Oral Medicine in Dermatology

Editors

ERIC T. STOOPLER
THOMAS P. SOLLECITO

DERMATOLOGIC CLINICS

www.derm.theclinics.com

Consulting Editor
BRUCE H. THIERS

October 2020 • Volume 38 • Number 4

ELSEVIER

1600 John F. Kennedy Boulevard • Suite 1800 • Philadelphia, Pennsylvania, 19103-2899

http://www.theclinics.com

DERMATOLOGIC CLINICS Volume 38, Number 4
October 2020 ISSN 0733-8635, ISBN-13: 978-0-323-75480-4

Editor: Lauren Boyle
Developmental Editor: Julia McKenzie

Dermatologic Clinics (ISSN 0733-8635) is published quarterly by Elsevier Inc., 360 Park Avenue South, New York, NY 10010-1710. Months of publication are January, April, July, and October. Business and editorial offices: 1600 John F. Kennedy Blvd., Suite 1800, Philadelphia, PA 19103-2899. Customer service office: 11830 Westline Drive, St. Louis, MO 63146. Periodicals postage paid at New York, NY, and additional mailing offices. Subscription prices are USD 408.00 per year for US individuals, USD 780.00 per year for US institutions, USD 456.00 per year for Canadian individuals, USD 952.00 per year for Canadian institutions, USD 510.00 per year for international individuals, USD 952.00 per year for international institutions, USD 100.00 per year for US students/residents, USD 100.00 per year for Canadian students/residents, and USD 240 per year for international students/residents. International air speed delivery is included in all *Clinics* subscription prices. All prices are subject to change without notice. **POSTMASTER:** Send address changes to *Dermatologic Clinics*, Elsevier Health Sciences Division, Subscription Customer Service, 3251 Riverport Lane, Maryland Heights, MO 63043. **Customer Service: 1-800-654-2452 (U.S. and Canada); 314-447-8871 (outside U.S. and Canada). Fax: 314-447-8029. E-mail: journalscustomerservice-usa@elsevier.com (for print support); journalsonlinesupport-usa@elsevier.com (for online support).**

Reprints. For copies of 100 or more, of articles in this publication, please contact the Commercial Reprints Department, Elsevier Inc., 360 Park Avenue South, New York, New York 10010-1710. Tel.: 212-633-3874; Fax: 212-633-3820; Email: reprints@elsevier.com.

The *Dermatologic Clinics* is covered in *MEDLINE/PubMed (Index Medicus)*, *Current Contents/Clinical Medicine*, *Excerpta Medica*, *Chemical Abstracts*, and *ISI/BIOMED*.

Contributors

CONSULTING EDITOR

BRUCE H. THIERS, MD
Professor and Chairman Emeritus, Department
of Dermatology and Dermatologic Surgery,
Medical University of South Carolina,
Charleston, South Carolina

EDITORS

**ERIC T. STOOPLER, DMD, FDSRCS,
FDSRCPS**
Professor, Department of Oral Medicine, Penn
Dental Medicine, Professor of Oral Medicine in
Medicine, Department of Medicine, Perelman
School of Medicine, University of
Pennsylvania, Philadelphia, Pennsylvania, USA

THOMAS P. SOLLECITO, DMD, FDS RCSEd
Chairman and Professor, Department of Oral
Medicine, Penn Dental Medicine, Chief, Oral

Medicine Division, Penn Medicine, Professor of
Oral Medicine in Medicine, Department of
Medicine, Professor of Oral Medicine in
Otorhinolaryngology: Head and Neck Surgery,
Department of OtorhinolaryngologyeHead and
Neck Surgery, Perelman School of Medicine,
University of Pennsylvania, Philadelphia,
Pennsylvania, USA

AUTHORS

SUNDAY O. AKINTOYE, BDS, DDS, MS
Associate Professor, Director of Oral Medicine
Research Program, Department of Oral
Medicine, University of Pennsylvania, School
of Dental Medicine, Philadelphia,
Pennsylvania, USA

FAIZAN ALAWI, DDS
Professor of Pathology, Department of Basic
and Translational Sciences, University of
Pennsylvania, School of Dental Medicine,
Philadelphia, Pennsylvania, USA

**MICHAEL T. BRENNAN, DDS, MHS,
FDSRCS(Ed)**
Professor and Chair, Department of Oral
Medicine, Atrium Health's Carolinas Medical
Center, Charlotte, North Carolina, USA

ALAA F. BUKHARI, BDS, MS
Assistant Professor, Oral Diagnostic Sciences
Department, Oral Medicine Division, King

Abdulaziz University, Faculty of Dentistry,
Jeddah, Saudi Arabia

KATHARINE CIARROCCA, DMD, MSEd
Associate Professor and Head of Oral
Medicine, Director of Interprofessional
Education, The University of North Carolina at
Chapel Hill, Adams School of Dentistry, Chapel
Hill, North Carolina, USA

GLEN H. CRAWFORD, MD, FAAD
Clinical Associate Professor, Department of
Dermatology, University of Pennsylvania,
Philadelphia, Pennsylvania, USA

SCOTT S. DE ROSSI, DMD, MBA
Dean and Professor, The University of North
Carolina at Chapel Hill, Adams School of
Dentistry, Chapel Hill, North Carolina, USA

BHAVIK DESAI, DMD, PhD
Private Practice, Affiliated Health of Wisconsin,
Milwaukee, Wisconsin, USA

SHARON ELAD, DMD, MSc
Professor and Chair, Division of Oral Medicine,
Principal Consultant, Hospital Dentistry,
Eastman Institute for Oral Health, University of
Rochester Medical Center, Rochester, New
York, USA

ARWA M. FARAG, BDS, DMSc
Assistant Professor, Oral Diagnostic Sciences
Department, Oral Medicine Division, King
Abdulaziz University, Faculty of Dentistry,
Jeddah, Saudi Arabia; Department of
Diagnostic Sciences, Division of Oral Medicine,
Tufts University School of Dental Medicine,
Boston, Massachusetts, USA

KATHERINE FRANCE, DMD, MBE
Assistant Professor of Oral Medicine,
University of Pennsylvania, School of Dental
Medicine, Philadelphia, Pennsylvania, USA

MICHAELL A. HUBER, DDS
Professor, University of Texas Health Science
Center San Antonio, School of Dentistry, San
Antonio, Texas, USA

ALEXANDER R. KERR, DDS, MSD
Clinical Professor, New York University College
of Dentistry, New York, New York, USA

BRITTANY KLEIN, DDS
Oral Medicine Resident PGY-1, Brigham and
Women's Hospital, Boston, Massachusetts,
USA

EUGENE KO, DDS
Clinical Assistant Professor, Diplomate of
American Oral and Maxillofacial Pathology,
Department of Oral Medicine, University of
Pennsylvania, School of Dental Medicine,
Philadelphia, Pennsylvania, USA

SATISH S. KUMAR, DMD, MDSc, MS
Associate Professor and Director, Periodontics,
Arizona School of Dentistry and Oral Health,
A.T. Still University, Mesa, Arizona, USA

JOEL M. LAUDENBACH, DMD
Associate Professor of Oral Medicine,
Carolinas Center for Oral Health - Atrium
Health, Charlotte, North Carolina, USA

MEL MUPPARAPU, DMD, MDS
Director of Radiology, Professor of Clinical Oral
Medicine, Department of Oral Medicine,

School of Dental Medicine, University of
Pennsylvania, Philadelphia, Pennsylvania, USA

JOEL J. NAPEÑAS, DDS, FDSRCS(Ed)
Associate Professor of Oral Medicine, Director,
Oral Medicine Residency Program,
Department of Oral Medicine, Atrium Health's
Carolinas Medical Center, Charlotte, North
Carolina, USA

DAVID OJEDA, DDS
Clinical Assistant Professor, University of
Texas Health Science Center San Antonio,
School of Dentistry, San Antonio, Texas, USA

TEMITOPE OMOLEHINWA, DMD
Assistant Professor, Department of Oral
Medicine, University of Pennsylvania, School
of Dental Medicine, Philadelphia,
Pennsylvania, USA

NEERAJ PANCHAL, DDS, MD, MA
Clinical Assistant Professor, Department of
Oral Surgery, University of Pennsylvania,
School of Dental Medicine, Philadelphia,
Pennsylvania, USA

JACOB P. REINHART, MD
US Navy, San Diego, California, USA

MISHA ROSENBACH, MD
Associate Professor, Department of
Dermatology, Hospital of the University of
Pennsylvania, Philadelphia, Pennsylvania, USA

RABIE M. SHANTI, DMD, MD
Assistant Professor of Otorhinolaryngology–
Head and Neck Surgery, Perelman School of
Medicine, University of Pennsylvania,
Philadelphia, Pennsylvania, USA

WESLEY SHERRELL, DMD
Assistant Professor, Oral Medicine, Division of
Diagnostic Sciences, The University of North
Carolina at Chapel Hill, Adams School of
Dentistry, Chapel Hill, North Carolina, USA

BRIDGET E. SHIELDS, MD
Medical Dermatology Fellow, Department of
Dermatology, Hospital of the University of
Pennsylvania, Philadelphia, Pennsylvania, USA

THOMAS P. SOLLECITO, DMD, FDS RCSEd
Chairman and Professor, Department of Oral
Medicine, Penn Dental Medicine, Chief, Oral

Medicine Division, Penn Medicine, Professor of Oral Medicine in Medicine, Department of Medicine, Professor of Oral Medicine in Otorhinolaryngology: Head and Neck Surgery, Department of OtorhinolaryngologyeHead and Neck Surgery, Perelman School of Medicine, University of Pennsylvania, Philadelphia, Pennsylvania, USA

DAVID C. STANTON, DMD, MD, FACS
Associate Professor, Oral and Maxillofacial Surgery, University of Pennsylvania Health System, Attending Surgeon, Oral and Maxillofacial Surgery, Children's Hospital of Philadelphia, Department of Oral and Maxillofacial Surgery, Perelman Center, Philadelphia, Pennsylvania, USA

ERIC T. STOOPLER, DMD, FDSRCS, FDSRCPS
Professor, Department of Oral Medicine, Penn Dental Medicine, Professor of Oral Medicine in Medicine, Department of Medicine, Perelman School of Medicine, University of Pennsylvania, Philadelphia, Pennsylvania, USA

TAKAKO TANAKA, DDS, FDS, RCSEd
Department of Oral Medicine, University of Pennsylvania, School of Dental Medicine, Philadelphia, Pennsylvania, USA

JAISRI R. THOPPAY, DDS, MBA, MS
President, Center for Integrative Oral Health Inc., Winter Park, Florida, USA

NATHANIEL S. TREISTER, DMD, DMSc
Associate Professor, Division of Oral and Maxillofacial Surgery, Oral Medicine and Dentistry, Brigham and Women's Hospital, Boston, Massachusetts, USA

ALESSANDRO VILLA, DDS, PhD, MPH
Chief, Oral Medicine, Associate Professor, Department of Orofacial Sciences, University of California, San Francisco, San Francisco, California, USA

SOOK-BIN WOO, DMD, MMSc
Associate Surgeon, Division of Oral Medicine and Dentistry, Brigham and Women's Hospital, Associate Professor, Department of Oral Medicine, Infection and Immunity, Harvard School of Dental Medicine, Boston, Massachusetts, USA

ANNA YUAN, DMD, PhD
Assistant Professor, Division of Oral Medicine, Tufts University School of Dental Medicine, Boston, Massachusetts, USA

Contents

Clinicians should be knowledgeable about the anatomy of the oral cavity and variations of normal because of oral and systemic health connections. This article presents an overview of normal and variations of normal anatomy of the oral cavity.

Oral health is a critical component of overall health and well-being. Dental caries and periodontitis are two of the most common oral diseases and, when not treated, can have irreversible sequelae and overall psychosocial and physiologic impact on individuals, diminishing quality of life. The burden of advanced dental caries and periodontal disease leading to tooth loss is severe. Physicians and allied medical professionals can help in early detection of dental caries, abscess, and periodontal diseases and initiate management followed by prompt referral to dental colleagues.

Squamous cell carcinoma makes up 90% of cases of oral cancer. However, a myriad of premalignant, inflammatory, and immune-based conditions can manifest as oral mucosal lesions. Biopsy of these lesions shares many of the principles of cutaneous lesions. Biopsy of oral mucosal lesions is a procedure that is safely performed in most cases in the outpatient ambulatory setting using local anesthesia. Special considerations should be taken depending on the presumed diagnosis based on physical examination. Its clinical relevance depends on a sound clinicopathologic assessment of the patient's condition. This article reviews specific considerations for biopsy of oral mucosal lesions.

Granulomatous diseases are chronic inflammatory disorders whose pathogenesis is triggered by an array of infectious and noninfectious agents, and may be localized or a manifestation of systemic, disseminated disease. As in the skin, oral manifestations of granulomatous inflammation are often nonspecific in their clinical appearance. Thus, in the absence of overt foreign material or a recognizable infectious agent, identifying the underlying cause of the inflammation can be challenging. This article highlights various conditions known to induce granulomatous inflammation within the oral soft tissues.

A variety of acute oral lesions may be encountered in the scope of dermatology. Oral lesions may be single or multiple; may arise secondary to infectious, immune, congenital, medication use, or idiopathic causes; and may take a variety of forms. A thorough evaluation of the oral cavity is required to assess patients with oral lesions. Affected patients may be monitored, treated, or referred to an appropriate specialist for further management as needed. Many acute oral lesions are self-limiting in nature and patients may require only assessment and reassurance. Several common acute oral lesions are discussed in this article.

Chronic oral mucosal lesions can be associated with several mucocutaneous diseases. This article reviews the autoimmune and immune-mediated, reactive, genetic, and infectious diseases that may present with chronic oral and/or cutaneous manifestations and provides a rational approach to diagnosis and management.

Allergic contact hypersensitivity reactions of the oral mucosa pose a significant medical concern for some patients. Oral hypersensitivity reactions can result from a vast number of allergenic chemicals, but occur commonly from dental materials, flavorings, and preservatives. Clinical presentation is varied and often overlaps with other oral conditions, complicating their diagnosis and management. The most common clinical entities associated with oral hypersensitivity reactions are oral lichenoid reactions and allergic contact cheilitis. In addition to reviewing these conditions and their most common corresponding allergens, this article summarizes the pathogenesis of oral hypersensitivity reactions and addresses patch testing pearls.

Burning mouth syndrome is a chronic condition characterized by an intraoral burning sensation in the absence of a local or systemic cause.

Oral pigmented lesions have a wide range of clinical presentations, some of which correlate with cutaneous pigmented lesions. This article highlights these correlates and underscores important differences that can potentially have clinical impact. Moreover, given a nonspecific presentation of an oral pigmented lesion, the article provides a reference to aid clinicians with differential diagnoses based on clinical features. This article is an overview of pigmented lesions of the oral cavity, including localized reactive pigmented lesions, neoplastic pigmented lesions, and pigmented lesions as sequelae of a systemic disease.

DERMATOLOGIC CLINICS

SERIES OF RELATED INTEREST

Immunology and Allergy Clinics of North America
Available at: http://www.immunology.theclinics.com/

THE CLINICS ARE AVAILABLE ONLINE!
Access your subscription at:
www.theclinics.com

Preface

Oral Medicine in Dermatology: An Interprofessional Partnership

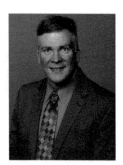
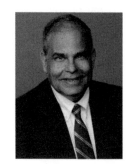

Eric T. Stoopler, DMD, FDSRCS, FDSRCPS   Thomas P. Sollecito, DMD, FDS RCSEd

Editors

Oral Medicine specialists are primarily concerned with the evaluation, diagnosis, and management of patients with oral mucosal diseases. In some cases, mucosal diseases may be limited to the oral cavity; however, it is common for patients to experience cutaneous manifestations of these conditions. The nature of these disorders necessitates a strong partnership between Oral Medicine and Dermatology. This issue of *Dermatologic Clinics*, entitled Oral Medicine in Dermatology, is designed to provide clinical information regarding health and disease of the oral cavity and perioral structures, with emphasis on relevance to the practicing dermatologist.

Dermatologists require knowledge of anatomical structures in the oral cavity and perioral region, so they are equipped to distinguish normal versus pathologic findings. Many benign conditions affecting these structures may appear pathologic, while significant pathologic conditions may be evocative of normal variants. Patients with acute and chronic mucosal diseases often initially consult with dermatologists. Patients may present with other oral complaints that mimic signs and symptoms of oral mucosal diseases that dermatologists must be familiar with, such as burning mouth syndrome. Oral counterparts of familiar dermatologic conditions, such as hypersensitivity reactions, pigmented lesions, and adverse drug reactions, may represent diagnostic and therapeutic challenges. The range of clinical presentation of oral premalignant disorders and oral cancer, a major cause of morbidity and mortality, is impressive, and recognition of the earliest clinical signs of this potentially devastating disease is critical. Many systemic diseases potentially affect and/or manifest in the oral and/or perioral areas. The oral cavity often provides a window to systemic health and may be the initial site of presentation of an underlying disease process. When a dermatologist evaluates the oral cavity and perioral structures, they must be aware that local oral disease may be present, or the oral condition may be a result of an underlying disorder that often requires further investigation. Finally, it is important for dermatologists to appreciate the challenges often associated with maintenance of oral hygiene and provision of dental care for patients with oral mucosal diseases.

All of the contributing authors have been carefully selected and are renowned clinicians, educators, and researchers in their respective fields. It is our hope that this issue provides valuable information to dermatologists in order to improve the quality of patient care for many years to come and to further substantiate the interprofessional relationship between dentistry and medicine.

Dedication

I dedicate this issue to my wife, Melanie, and my children, Ryan and Ethan, for their unconditional love, encouragement, and support of my academic endeavors. I also acknowledge and thank all of my mentors, colleagues, residents, students,

Dermatol Clin 38 (2020) xi–xii
https://doi.org/10.1016/j.det.2020.06.001
0733-8635/20/© 2020 Published by Elsevier Inc.

and patients, who have contributed to my professional development.

Eric T. Stoopler, DMD, FDSRCS, FDSRCPS

I dedicate this issue to my wife, Carolyn, and my children, Elizabeth, Peter, and Katharine, for their unconditional love and for their support of my academic pursuits. I also wish to acknowledge my mentors, colleagues, residents, students, and patients, who continually contribute to my professional development.

Thomas P. Sollecito, DMD, FDS, RCSEd

Eric T. Stoopler, DMD, FDSRCS, FDSRCPS
Department of Oral Medicine
Penn Dental Medicine
240 South 40th Street
Philadelphia, PA 19104, USA

Thomas P. Sollecito, DMD, FDS RCSEd
Department of Oral Medicine
Penn Dental Medicine
240 South 40th Street
Philadelphia, PA 19104, USA

E-mail addresses:
ets@upenn.edu (E.T. Stoopler)
tps@upenn.edu (T.P. Sollecito)

Clinical Evaluation and Anatomic Variation of the Oral Cavity

Sunday O. Akintoye, BDS, DDS, MS[a],*, Mel Mupparapu, DMD, MDS[b]

KEYWORDS

• Oral cavity • Mucosa • Lip • Tongue • Exostosis • Lymphoid • Leukodema • Fordyce granules

KEY POINTS

- Clinical evaluation of the oral cavity should include a thorough assessment of the soft and hard tissues.
- Distinguishing between normal and abnormal anatomic features in the oral cavity is vital to early diagnosis of oral pathologic conditions.
- Normal anatomic variations may mimic pathology.
- Periodic observation or follow up may be needed for certain anatomic variations.
- When symptomatic, these anatomic variations or abnormalities can be medically or surgically treated to relieve the symptoms.

INTRODUCTION

Evidence-based guidelines continue to point to a strong correlation between oral health and systemic diseases,[1,2] so health care providers should be knowledgeable regarding normal anatomy of the oral cavity and clinical implications of abnormal findings. Clinical evaluation of the oral cavity should start with the assessment of the head, face, and neck regions. It is important to identify any asymmetry or changes caused by abnormalities of the salivary glands, head and neck lymph nodes, and cranial nerves as well as changes in the skull size and shape.

In addition, any changes in skin color, abnormal pigmentation, and hairline distribution could be an indication of pathologic conditions that warrant further investigation. This article presents an overview of anatomy, as well as anatomic variations often encountered during a clinical evaluation.

ANATOMY AND CLINICAL EVALUATION TECHNIQUES

Extraoral Region

Evaluation of the extraoral region starts with a visual inspection to confirm the symmetric features of the facial appearance and identify any obvious deviation from normal. The right and left halves of the face are usually mirror images of each other so any asymmetry caused by disorder or facial palsy should be readily identified. Abnormal swellings of the major salivary glands and lymph nodes that may not be obvious during visual inspection may be better appreciated by palpation of the right and left sides of the head, face, and neck simultaneously to compare both sides. The inspection of the neck should rule out any scarring, masses, or the presence of torticollis. Cervical lymphadenopathy can be ruled out by palpation of the lymph nodes. Tracheal position should be inspected for deviation from either a neck mass or more serious conditions such as pneumothorax. The thyroid

[a] Department of Oral Medicine, School of Dental Medicine, University of Pennsylvania, 240 South 40th Street Suite 211, Philadelphia, PA 19104, USA; [b] Department of Oral Medicine, School of Dental Medicine, University of Pennsylvania, 240 South 40th Street Suite 214, Philadelphia, PA 19104, USA
* Corresponding author.
E-mail address: akintoye@upenn.edu

Dermatol Clin 38 (2020) 399–411
https://doi.org/10.1016/j.det.2020.05.001

gland should be inspected at both rest and as the patient swallows for goiters or nodules. If positioned behind the patient, the thyroid gland can be palpated for identification of the isthmus and the lateral lobes, both at rest and as the patient swallows, to be able to identify goiter, nodule, or thyroiditis. Cranial nerve II to XII function should be generally assessed. The presence of any abnormal findings often indicates the need to critically evaluate for any associated or corroborating intraoral abnormal features during the intraoral evaluation.

Oral Region

The anatomic structures in the oral region of the head and neck include the lips, oral cavity proper, palate, tongue, floor of mouth, and oropharynx (**Fig. 1**). The mouth or oral cavity is the gateway to the body through the gastrointestinal tract. It consists of unique structures that perform many functions essential for life. These functions include mastication, speech, respiration, digestion, swallowing, and taste.

The processing and digestion of food start with a well-functioning oral soft and hard tissues and salivation.[3,4] Poor nutrition heightens the chances of poor oral health.[5] Several aging changes and medication side effects that diminish appetite, taste, and smell sensitivities, and oral mucosal properties, can affect nutritional status and often become evident in the oral cavity.[6]

Oral cavity

The oral cavity consists of the vestibule and oral cavity proper. The vestibule is the space between the teeth and the mucosa of the lips and cheeks (see **Fig. 1**). The vestibule is bounded medially by the teeth and its anterior and lateral boundaries are the intraoral mucosal surfaces of the lips and cheeks. The vestibule gradually narrows posteriorly as the medial and lateral boundaries converge at the retromolar region, which is the region of the oral cavity posterior to the last mandibular and maxillary molar teeth. However, the oral cavity proper is the space in the interior of the mouth between the upper and lower dental arches occupied by the tongue when the mouth is closed or at rest (see **Fig. 1**). The teeth and alveolar bone on the left and right sides separate the vestibule on each side from the oral cavity proper. The oral cavity proper is bounded anteriorly and laterally by the lingual surfaces of the teeth and alveolar processes on the left and right sides of the mouth (see **Fig. 1**). The circumoral facial muscles control the opening of the mouth vestibule and the muscles of mastication control movement of the mandible. The posterior limit of the oral cavity is the oropharynx

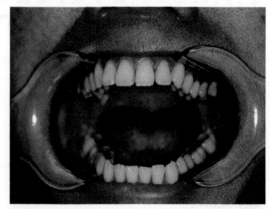

Fig. 1. Oral cavity. The oral cavity showing the space in the interior of the mouth between the upper and lower dental arches with their respective maxillary and mandibular teeth.

and the palatoglossal arches bordering the oropharynx on each side. Superiorly, the oral cavity is separated from the nasal cavity by the hard and soft palates. Inferiorly, the mylohyoid muscle extends from the left and right mandible to support the tongue and floor of the mouth. The terminologies used to describe different areas of the oral cavity are based on their relationship to the tongue within the oral cavity proper, the palate, cheek, facial surface, or lips, which all define the boundaries of the oral cavity. Hence, the term lingual describes a structure closest to the tongue, palatal and buccal describe the ones closest to the palate or inner cheek respectively, and facial or labial are used to describe structures closest to the facial surface or lips, respectively.

Lips and cheeks

Visual inspection and palpation of the upper and lower lips, the muscular folds that surround the entrance of the mouth, is important (**Fig. 2**). This inspection allows assessment of color changes, firmness, and presence or absence of any unusual

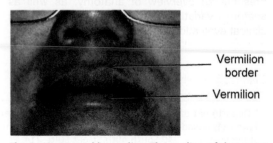

_____ Vermilion border

_____ Vermilion

Fig. 2. Upper and lower lips. The outline of the upper and lower lips showing the distinct vermilion zone and vermilion border where the skin of the external aspect of the lips terminates.

nodules. The skin of the external aspect of the lip terminates at the vermilion border, which marks the beginning of transition to the vermilion zone. The darker appearance of the vermilion zone relative to the surrounding skin is caused by the underlying blood vessels beneath the thin surface epithelium. The vermilion zone gradually blends intraorally with the oral mucosa (see **Fig. 2**). During a visual inspection, it should be noted that the width of both lips is usually within the distance between the irises of the eyes. The philtrum, a midline vertical groove on the upper lip, extends from the nasal septum to the tubercle region of the upper lip, making it easy to identify asymmetry in a patient's appearance. Palpation of the lips is best achieved by pulling out each lip slightly and palpating it bidigitally both extraorally and intraorally (**Fig. 3**).

Oral mucosa

The oral cavity mucous membrane, referred to as mucosa, is named and identified based on its location within the oral cavity. On histology, the oral mucosa is made up of stratified squamous epithelium that may or may not be keratinized, depending on the region of the oral cavity. The labial mucosa lines the inner portions of the lip, whereas the buccal mucosa lines the inner portion of the cheeks (see **Fig. 3**; **Fig. 4**). Intraorally, the labial mucosa terminates at the vestibular fold as it gradually reflects onto the alveolar bone supporting the anterior teeth. The anterior vestibular fold, known as the mucolabial fold, extends posteriorly

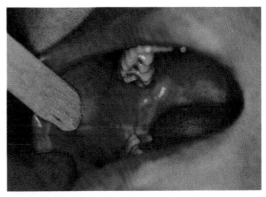

Fig. 4. Evaluation of the buccal mucosa. Assessment of the buccal mucosa and mucobuccal vestibular fold can be facilitated by using a wooden spatula or dental mouth mirror to retract the cheeks.

on the left and right sides of the oral cavity as the mucobuccal fold to distinguish where the buccal mucosa reflects onto the alveolar bone, which supports the posterior teeth. The mucous membrane that covers the alveolar bone, in which the roots of the teeth are anchored, is referred to as alveolar mucosa. To thoroughly examine the buccal mucosa, the patient should be asked to open the mouth slightly and the lips and cheeks pulled away gently from the teeth with a wooden spatula or dental mouth mirror if available (see **Figs. 3** and **4**). Bidigital palpation and circumferential compression with 1 finger on the cheek extraorally and another finger intraorally on the buccal mucosa makes it easy to identify any mass within the soft tissues.

Gingivae

The oral mucosa terminates around the teeth as gingiva that surrounds the maxillary and mandibular teeth (**Fig. 5**). The nonattached, scallop-shaped marginal gingiva covers the roots of teeth anchored within the alveolar bone. The marginal

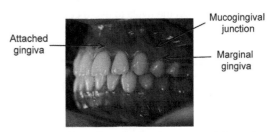

Fig. 5. Gingiva. The gingiva is separated into the scallop-shaped nonattached marginal gingiva and the attached gingiva tightly adherent to the alveolar bone. The mucogingival junction demarcates the transition zone between the attached gingiva and alveolar mucosa.

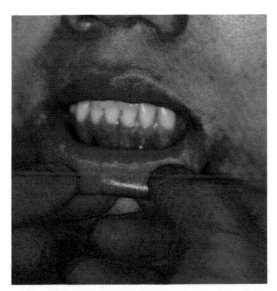

Fig. 3. Evaluation of the lips. Assessment of the lips is best achieved by pulling each lip slightly to palpate its extraoral and intraoral surfaces.

gingiva wedged between adjacent teeth is the interdental gingiva or papillae. The inner surface of the marginal gingiva that juxtaposes the tooth surface harbors a space called the sulcus or crevice filled with saliva, known as crevicular fluid. The marginal gingiva extends as the firm attached gingiva that is tightly adherent to the alveolar bone surrounding the roots of the teeth (see **Fig. 5**). Often the attached gingiva has regions of pigmentation that are dictated by race or ethnicity. It is common for African people and dark-skinned individuals to have attached gingiva that is darker than the surrounding oral mucosa. This condition should be distinguished from so-called beauty tattoos, which are common in some ethnic groups, and amalgam tattoo, which can occur because of inadvertent impregnation of amalgam particles into the gingiva during a dental procedure. The demarcation between the attached gingiva and the loose, slightly more movable alveolar mucosa is the mucogingival junction.

Palate

A visual examination of the palate reveals that the palatal mucosa extends laterally on the left and right to the palatal gingiva overlying the maxillary arch in the oral cavity. The mucosa of the anterior hard palate is dense, firmly attached to the underlying palatal bone, and has distinct parallel transverse mucosal ridges or palatal rugae (**Fig. 6**). The median palatal raphe is a midline ridge of tissue that bisects the hard palate into 2 equal left and right regions. The soft palate occupies the posterior third of the palate. It has a smooth and movable mucosa because it does not have any bone support like the hard palate. Its posterior free edge ends in a midline pendulous projection called the uvula (**Fig. 7**). On either side of the uvula are the anterior and posterior arches forming the palatoglossus and palatopharyngeal arches. The palatal tonsils, a mass of lymphoid tissue, is positioned between the 2 arches. The hard and soft palates can be readily palpated but it is advisable to visually inspect the uvula to avoid causing a gag reflex. This inspection can be achieved by gently depressing the tongue with a wooden tongue depressor while asking the patient to say "Ah" to observe a slight anteroposterior movement of the uvula and a more conspicuous view of the pharyngeal arches.

Tongue

When describing the tongue, the terms dorsal and ventral are not synonymous with posterior and anterior respectively because all are descriptive terms that separately apply to the tongue. The bulk of the tongue is the highly mobile anterior

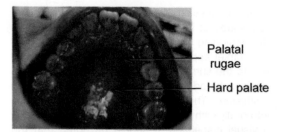

Fig. 6. Palate. The hard palate showing distinct parallel transverse mucosal ridges or rugae.

two-thirds, or the body of the tongue, which resides in the oral cavity and is readily visible when protruded (**Fig. 8**A). The posterior third of the tongue, or base of the tongue, is less mobile because is attached to the floor of the mouth and extends down into the pharynx. Most of the tongue base is usually not visible during a routine examination. The ventral surface of the tongue is in contact with the floor of the mouth, whereas the top or dorsal surface is covered with many lingual papillae (see **Fig. 8**A). A midline median sulcus on the dorsum of the tongue runs posteriorly from the apex or tip of the tongue. It bisects the tongue into 2 equal halves so, during a clinical evaluation, it is possible to identify any asymmetry and the location of any variations, abnormality, or lesions caused by a disorder. The dorsum of the tongue has slender, threadlike filiform lingual papillae that can be readily differentiated from the red mushroom-shaped fungiform lingual papillae. The tongue should be carefully examined by grasping and pulling it forward with a piece of gauze pad wrapped around the anterior third to get a firm grip (**Fig. 8**B). Further posteriorly, an inverted V-shaped groove with the tip pointing posteriorly toward the pharynx, called sulcus

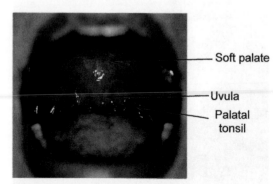

Fig. 7. Soft palate and uvula. The soft palate showing the uvula at the midline of the posterior edge. On either side of the uvula are the anterior and posterior arches forming the palatoglossus and palatopharyngeal arches.

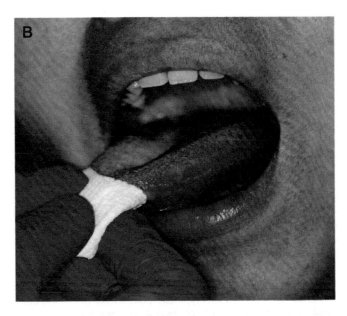

Fig. 8. Dorsal (A) and ventral (B) tongue and grasping of tongue with gauze. The tongue is best assessed by grasping and pulling it forward with a piece of gauze pad wrapped around the anterior third to get a firm grip.

terminalis, is visible at the intersection of the anterior two-thirds and posterior third of the tongue. Lining the anterior side of the sulcus terminalis are the larger mushroom-shaped circumvallate lingual papillae (Fig. 9). Note that the tip of the inverted V pattern has a small, pitlike depression known as foramen cecum. If the tongue is pulled further forward, the irregular mass of tonsillar tissue, the lingual tonsil, will be visible. This mass is different from the palatine tonsils on either side of the uvula between the palatoglossus and palatopharyngeal arches. Foliate lingual papillae are bilaterally symmetric areas of pinkish-red vertical folds or grooves located in the posterior part of the lateral borders of the tongue. They are located anterior to the circumvallate papillae. The foliate lingual papillae are vestigial in humans and should not be confused with an abnormal tongue lesion. Foliate lingual papillae appear brighter red than the surrounding lingual mucosa, and contain taste buds and lymphoid tissues. Lingual tonsils can become enlarged if traumatized or during upper respiratory tract infections. The corresponding

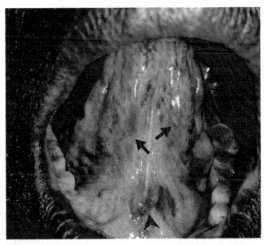

Fig. 10. Ventral tongue. Black arrows point to the prominent lingual nerves bilaterally on the ventral surface of the tongue, and the black arrowhead points to the sublingual caruncle through which the submandibular and sublingual salivary glands secrete saliva into the floor of the mouth.

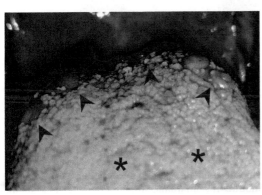

Fig. 9. Circumvallate lingual papillae. Black arrowheads point to the mushroom-shaped circumvallate lingual papillae and the black stars indicate the excessive coating on the dorsum of the tongue.

enlargement of the foliate papillae is referred to as transient lingual papillitis.[7,8] Both foliate papillae and lingual tonsils are normal anatomic structures and no treatment is indicated for their enlargement because the condition is transient. Although the tongue is still gently pulled forward during an oral evaluation, the lateral borders of the tongue should also be examined for any mucosal or papillary changes. An evaluation of the tongue should conclude by asking the patient to raise the tongue to inspect the ventral or sublingual surface (**Fig. 10**). The sublingual mucosa is thin, shiny, and transparent, disclosing numerous blood vessels, especially the 2 large, deep lingual veins that run parallel on either side of the tongue midline. Lateral to each lingual vein are folds of fingerlike projections called plica fimbriata.

Lymphoid aggregates

Lymphoid aggregates are typically collections of focal hyperplastic lymphoid tissue or normal lymphoid tissue that may occur anywhere in the oral cavity (see **Fig. 7**). They are commonly seen in the region of the Waldeyer tonsillar ring, which includes the floor of the mouth, soft palate, lateral border of the tongue, and oropharynx. Lymphoid tissue on the lateral wall of the oropharynx around the opening of the eustachian tube is referred to as tubal tonsils. The combination of the palatine tonsils, lingual tonsils, and tubal tonsils complete the Waldeyer tonsillar ring. Lymphoid tissue aggregates within the mucosa of the roof of the nasopharynx are collectively referred to as the pharyngeal tonsil. These aggregates are located in the midline and form the superior aspect of the Waldeyer tonsillar ring. The lymphoid aggregates, when enlarged, are referred to as adenoids.

Floor of mouth

The floor of the mouth is inferior to the ventral surface of the tongue. It is bounded by the mylohyoid muscle inferiorly, the medial surface of the right and left mandibular body, and superiorly by a thin mucosal layer that is continuous with the mucous membrane of the ventral tongue. Beneath the thin mucosa of the floor of the mouth are several blood vessels, nerves, ganglia, and 2 major salivary glands on either side of the midline: the sublingual and submandibular salivary glands. Also note that the lingual nerve, which is the terminal branch of the mandibular nerve, has a variable course in its relationship to the mandibular alveolar crest, submandibular salivary gland duct, and floor of the mouth. It innervates the mucous membrane of the anterior two-thirds of the tongue, floor of oral cavity, and the adjacent lingual gingiva. The lingual frenum is a midline fold of tissue that runs from the

ventral surface of the tongue, bisecting the floor of the mouth and terminating on the lingual gingiva between the 2 mandibular central incisors. On either side of the lingual frenum are the sublingual caruncle, the papillae that contain the openings of the ducts of the submandibular salivary glands. Also, conspicuously visible on the floor of the mouth is a horseshoe-shaped swelling, the sublingual fold or ridge caused by the underlying sublingual salivary glands. The sublingual fold has multiple ductal openings of the sublingual salivary gland. Some of these ducts also merge with the submandibular salivary gland duct to secrete saliva into the floor of the mouth at the sublingual caruncle (see **Fig. 10**). The floor of the mouth should be assessed by bimanual palpation. This palpation is done by placing the index finger of 1 hand intraorally in the floor of the mouth and 1 or 2 fingertips of the opposite hand extraorally under the chin (**Fig. 11**). By compressing the tissues between the fingers, it is possible to compare the right and left sides of the floor of the mouth and feel for any unusual nodule. If the sublingual caruncle is carefully dried with a piece of gauze swab, the submandibular and sublingual salivary glands can be compressed to observe salivary flow from the ductal orifices.

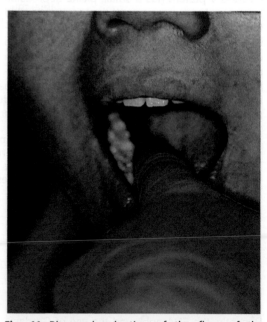

Fig. 11. Bimanual palpation of the floor of the mouth. The anatomic structures in the floor of the mouth assessed by bimanual palpation. Note the index finger of 1 hand intraorally in the floor of the mouth and 1 or 2 fingertips of the opposite hand placed extraorally under the chin.

Teeth

It is more practicable to examine the teeth with the appropriate dental instruments, which include a dental mouth mirror and dental explorer. However, dental arches in which the teeth are anchored can be divided into 4 quadrants: right and left maxillary and right and left mandibular quadrants (see **Fig. 1**). Adults have a total of 32 teeth, so each quadrant with full complements of permanent teeth should contain 2 incisors, 1 canine, 2 premolars, and 3 molars. However, children before the age of 6 years have a total of 20 teeth and each quadrant of the dental arch with full complements of deciduous teeth should contain 2 incisors, 1 canine, and 2 molars. Several terms are applicable when describing each tooth. The crown is the exposed part of the tooth in the oral cavity, whereas the root is the part anchored in the alveolar bone. The crown of each tooth has multiple surfaces. The occlusal surface of the crown refers to the masticating or biting surface; the vestibular surface of the crown, which faces the vestibule, is identified as the buccal surface if it is on a posterior tooth facing the cheek or the labial surface if it is on an anterior tooth facing the lips. The lingual surface faces the tongue, the mesial surface is the side of the crown closest to the patient's midline, whereas the distal surface is the side of the crown farthest from the midline.

Salivary glands and saliva

A thorough clinical evaluation of the oral cavity should also include palpation of the major salivary glands. The ducts of the paired parotid glands located in the preauricular and infra-auricular regions open intraorally in the buccal mucosa opposite the second maxillary molar tooth. By gently palpating and expressing the glands, flow of saliva from the parotid glands can be assessed intraorally by observing the secretions at the ductal openings. Bimanual digital palpation is the best way to "milk" the submandibular and sublingual salivary glands while observing the salivary flow from their ductal orifices at the floor of the mouth (see **Figs. 10** and **11**). The quantity of saliva based on flow and quality based on its organic and inorganic components are essential for the multiple functions of saliva.[7] Individuals with reduced salivary flow are susceptible to different oral disorders. Hyposalivation or decreased salivary flow can cause increase in oral microbial load, making oral mucosa susceptible to candidal infections, and the teeth are also at higher risks of developing dental caries. Xerostomia is a complaint of dry mouth caused by hyposalivation. Symptoms of dry mouth vary from individual to individual, so patients should always be asked whether they think that the amount of saliva in their mouth is enough, too little, or too much. This step is one of the first in identifying individuals with hyposalivation.

ANATOMIC VARIATIONS
Extraoral

Lip pits

Lip pits are developmental anomalies occurring commonly on the vermilion border of the lower lip, although they can also occur on the upper lip and the commissures or angles of the mouth (**Fig. 12**). The lip pits are also associated with a rare autosomal dominant syndrome called van der Woude syndrome, where lip pits occur independently or in association with cleft lip/cleft palate.[9] The prevalence of van der Woude syndrome ranges from 1 in 75,000 to 1 in 100,000 live births. Cleft lip with or without cleft palate occurs in about 70% of patients with van der Woude syndrome. Associated findings in this syndrome include hypodontia, club foot, syndactyly of hands, and genitourinary and cardiovascular abnormalities. Studies have identified abnormal chromosome band 1q32-q41 and 1p34 in patients affected with the van der Woude syndrome.[10] The lower lip pits can occur bilaterally and can be shallow or deep depending on the degree of gene expression. The pits sometimes connect to the orbicularis oris muscle and, if deep enough, can develop to a fistula. Occasionally, the pits penetrate the minor and accessory salivary glands located in the lips, resulting in salivary secretion from the pits. Genetic evaluation and

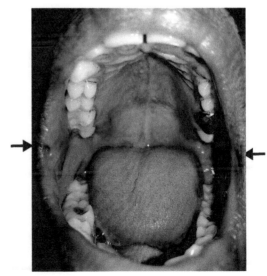

Fig. 12. Bilateral commissural lip pits. Lip pits (*arrows*) are common developmental anomalies that may occur in the vermilion border or the angles of the mouth.

counseling are recommended for patients with congenital lip pits and, if clinically indicated, surgical excision is the treatment of choice.[9]

Venous lakes

Venous lakes are benign pigmentations caused by dilated veins that are small. Typically seen in adults, these lesions are also known as phlebectases. They present as small, bluish-purple, slightly elevated soft tissue lesions that are noticeable on the exposed skin. The most common occurrence is reported in the face, lips, and the helix of the ears. The diagnosis of venous lakes is almost exclusively by appearance. On pressing, the color of the venous lake macule or papule disappears as the blood is cleared from the site. This finding is pathognomonic of this condition. A glass slide or the lens of a dermatoscope can be used to elicit this sign.

Sulci labiorum (lip prints)

The pattern of wrinkles (lip prints) on the upper and lower lips is unique to each individual[11,12] (**Fig. 13**). Evaluation of lip prints relative to the surrounding anatomy has been found to be stable and recordable, and classification of lip prints (**Table 1**) contributes to the armamentaria used in forensic sciences.[13]

Intraoral

Fordyce granules

Fordyce granules are commonly noted variations of normal anatomy within the oral mucosa. They

Table 1 Classification of lip prints	
Type I & I'	A clear-cut line or groove running vertically across the lip, or straight grooves that disappear halfway into the lip instead of covering the entire breadth of the lip or partial-length groove of type I
Type II	Grooves that fork in their course, or a branched groove
Type III	An intersected groove
Type IV	A reticular groove
Type V	Grooves that are not in any of the above categories and cannot be differentiated morphologically

Data from Andreeva VA, Kesse-Guyot E, Galan P, et al. Adherence to National Dietary Guidelines in Association with Oral Health Impact on Quality of Life. Nutrients 2018;10(5); and Solemdal K, Sandvik L, Willumsen T, et al. The impact of oral health on taste ability in acutely hospitalized elderly. PLoS One 2012;7(5):e36557.

are ectopic sebaceous glands trapped within the skin or epithelium that occurs in more than 80% of adults.[14] Sebaceous glands are part of normal skin in association with hair follicles. However, they present intraorally as yellowish-white papular areas of about 1 to 2 mm in diameter scattered

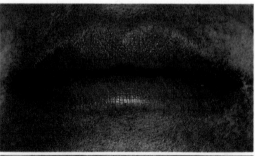
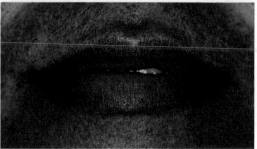

Fig. 13. Individual variations of lip prints. The vermilion zone of the lips display distinct pattern of wrinkles or prints unique to each individual.

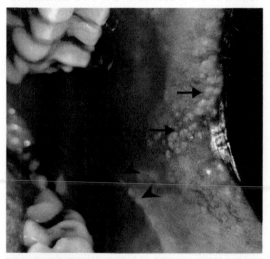

Fig. 14. Fordyce granules. Black arrows point to ectopic sebaceous glands trapped within the epithelium of the buccal mucosa presenting as Fordyce granules. Black arrowheads identify the linea alba buccalis on the buccal mucosa.

throughout the oral mucosa. They can be identified in the buccal mucosa bilaterally (**Fig. 14**) and on the vermilion of the upper lip. Fordyce granule seem to become more visible in the oral cavity after puberty because of hormonal changes, and their number is thought to increase with age.[14] Fordyce granules are asymptomatic and treatment is not necessary. On rare occasions if a biopsy is performed on an unusual presenting sebaceous gland, pseudocysts, sebaceous cell hyperplasia, and adenomas have been reported after a biopsy.[15] Fordyce granules can also mimic the appearance of pseudomembranous candidiasis, but candida plaques can be easily removed, whereas the Fordyce granules do not wipe off.

Lingual varicosities

Varicosities are abnormally dilated veins that are commonly seen in the elderly. Although they can be seen on any location, the most common locations are lips, buccal and labial mucosa, and ventral portion of the tongue (**Fig. 15**). It is thought that the varicosities are formed because of weakening of the vessel wall secondary to aging. Because they are variations of normal anatomy, no treatment is necessary except for esthetic reasons. The lesions become thrombosed on occasion.[16] On sites such as the lips, the varicosities may mimic mucoceles.

Leukoedema

Leukodema is a benign grayish-white appearance and often involves the buccal mucosa. It is an incidental finding during intraoral examination. Leukodema is characterized by the accumulation of fluid within the epithelial cells of buccal mucosa. It presents clinically as a white transparent mucosal alteration located bilaterally in the buccal mucosa with crisscrossing folds or lines within the area.[14] It is more common in men and less common in the white population. A distinguishing feature of leukodema is the clinical stretch test because it disappears when the mucosa is stretched. The differential diagnosis of this benign clinical entity includes white spongy nevus, frictional keratosis, Darier disease, pachyonychia congenita, candidiasis, lichen planus, and benign intraepithelial dyskeratosis.[17] There is no known relationship between leukoedema and dysplasia, and no treatment is necessary for leukodema because it is a variation of normal anatomy.

Exostosis: maxillary and mandibular tori and variations

Tori, also known as exostosis, are benign dense cortical nodular osseous structures. They may be located in the midline of the hard palate (torus palatinus) or bilaterally in the posterior maxillary

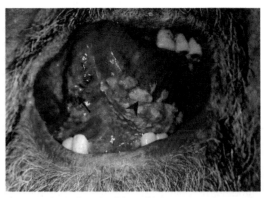

Fig. 15. Lingual varicosities. Black arrow points to the prominent dilated lingual vein or varicosity of the right side but obscured by a white lesion on the left side shown by black arrowhead.

molar regions along the buccal and palatal bony shelves (torus maxillaris), which may extend to the region of the maxillary tuberosity. They can also be located bilaterally along the lingual cortical plate of the mandible (torus mandibularis) (**Fig. 16**) or isolated beneath the labial and buccal alveolar mucosa (exostoses).

Because of the thin oral mucosa overlying the bony exostoses, tori appear as pale yellowish white because of the color of the underlying bone. Although these are distinct entities, clinicians must be careful to distinguish them from the bony expansions associated with other dentoalveolar disorders, such as fibrous dysplasia, cemento-osseous dysplasia, or Paget disease. No treatment is necessary unless it is clinically indicated to perform surgical recontouring before prosthodontic treatment.

Benign migratory glossitis (geographic tongue)

Benign migratory glossitis, or erythema migrans, is also commonly known as geographic tongue. This

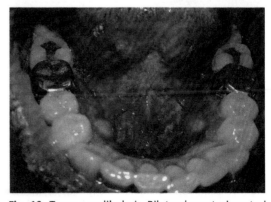

Fig. 16. Torus mandibularis. Bilateral exostosis or tori on the lingual surface of the mandible (*black arrows*), which are dense cortical nodular osseous swellings.

condition is characterized by red, erythematous regions of the dorsal and lateral borders of the anterior two-thirds of the tongue. The prevalence of geographic tongue is about 2% to 3% in the general population.[18] This condition features well-demarcated red areas caused by atrophy of the filiform papillae. The erythematous zones are more conspicuous because they are either partially or completely surrounded by a slightly elevated white scalloped or serpentine border (**Fig. 17**).[14] During the healing phase, the peripheral zone is the first to disappear, followed by healing of the red zone.

On histology, geographic tongue is characterized by hyperkeratosis and acanthosis resembling psoriasis. Therefore, some investigators consider it to be a form of intraoral psoriasis.[19] Geographic tongue is usually asymptomatic and no treatment is required. Some patients complain of burning sensation or increased sensitivity to hot or spicy foods. Topical steroids and or anesthetic agents along with reassurance is the treatment of choice.

Morsicatio buccarum (oral frictional hyperkeratosis)

Morsicatio buccarum, or cheek biting, is often noted in patient with compulsive neurosis (**Fig. 18**). The patient bites off pieces of the buccal mucous membrane, leading to excessive hyperkeratosis.[20] The typical location of hyperkeratosis in patients with morsicatio buccarum is along the line of the occlusal plane of the teeth, signifying the contact between upper and lower teeth. The mucobuccal folds are not affected by the trauma. The inner lip may also be irritated and traumatized

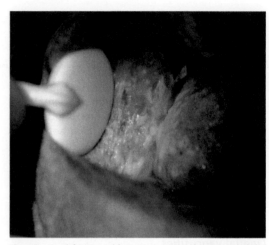

Fig. 18. Oral frictional keratosis. Hyperkeratosis of the buccal mucosa caused by trauma from habitual cheek biting.

by the anterior teeth, and this is known as morsicatio labiorum. A biopsy and microscopic assessment can be used to differentiate morsicatio from linea alba buccalis and white spongy nevus.

Linea alba buccalis

Line alba buccalis is a whitish-gray horizontal line on the buccal mucosa that is oriented parallel to the occlusal plane of the teeth (**Fig. 19**). It usually presents bilaterally in the oral cavity as a hyperkeratotic response to physiologic function, where the negative pressure pulls the buccal mucosa toward

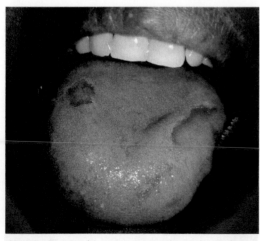

Fig. 17. Geographic tongue. Patchy red, erythematous regions on the dorsal and lateral borders of the anterior two-thirds of the tongue characterize geographic tongue.

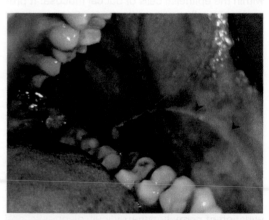

Fig. 19. Prominent linea alba buccalis on the left cheek mucosa. Whitish-gray hyperkeratotic horizontal line (*arrowheads*) on the buccal mucosa oriented parallel to the occlusal plane of the teeth. This condition is caused by repetitive negative pressure that pulls and attaches the buccal mucosa onto the buccal surfaces of the teeth leaving a keratotic line along the occlusal plane.

the teeth, causing a hyperkeratotic response. Linea alba buccalis is present in the oral cavity in about 13% of population and needs no treatment.[21]

Common oral disorders

Ankyloglossia Ankyloglossia is a developmental anomaly of the tongue characterized by an abnormally short, thick lingual frenum resulting in limitation of tongue movement. Complete ankyloglossia occurs when a short lingual frenum extends to the tip of the tongue causing restricted tongue movement. Most cases of ankyloglossia are partial ankyloglossia where the tip of the tongue has movement and flexibility but the tongue itself has some restricted movement (**Fig. 20**). Babies with ankyloglossia have difficulty with suckling during breastfeeding and adults may develop phonation and speech difficulties.[22]

Hairy tongue (lingua villosa nigra) Hairy tongue, sometimes also called black hairy tongue, is a benign condition characterized by elongation of the filiform papillae with a typical carpetlike presentation on the dorsum of the tongue. Predisposing factors are smoking, excessive coffee or black tea consumption, poor oral hygiene, general debilitation, xerostomia, and polypharmacy. Hairy tongue can also appear brown, green, blue, or nonpigmented. Black hairy tongue is generally asymptomatic but may be associated with halitosis, metallic taste, dysgeusia, burning mouth, and gagging.

Fissured tongue When the dorsal surface of tongue shows multiple small grooves or fissures,

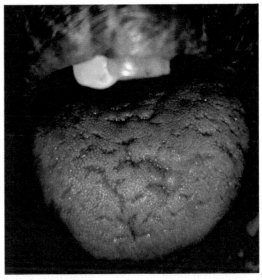

Fig. 21. Fissured or scrotal tongue. Dorsal surface of the tongue displaying multiple small shallow and deep grooves or fissures.

the condition is termed fissured tongue. The fissures can be single or multiple, shallow or deep, and occur commonly in the anterior two-thirds of the tongue (**Fig. 21**). Other terms used to describe fissured tongue include scrotal tongue, plicated tongue, and lingua plicata. The cause of fissured tongue is unknown. No treatment is necessary but the patient is encouraged to clean the surface of the tongue, preferably with a toothbrush, to prevent food debris from getting trapped within the

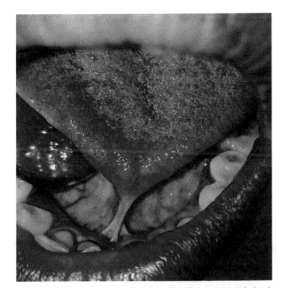

Fig. 20. Ankyloglossia. An abnormally short and thick lingual frenum restricting tongue movement.

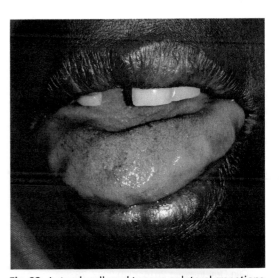

Fig. 22. Lateral scalloped tongue or lateral crenations. Tongue displaying scalloped or crenated margins often caused by pressure on an enlarged tongue by the surrounding teeth.

fissures. This cleaning prevents halitosis, tissue irritation, and even inflammation.[23]

Crenations of tongue (scalloped tongue) Crenated or scalloped tongue is a variation of normal tongue appearance caused by a combination of factors that include the size of the tongue, size of the teeth, status of existing dentition, and the pressure applied on the tongue by the surrounding teeth (**Fig. 22**). An enlarged tongue (macroglossia) can be a developmental anomaly, as often seen in Down syndrome, or secondary to systemic conditions such as hypothyroidism, sarcoidosis, and amyloidosis. A case of generalized lymphangioma was reported where macroglossia necessitated partial glossectomy. There is no specific treatment other than identifying sharp edges of teeth that have developed severe attrition or erosion and smoothening these off to prevent traumatic ulceration of the tongue.

SUMMARY

This article provides an overview of normal oral cavity anatomy within the context of variations of normal. It is vital that clinical evaluation of the oral cavity should include assessment of all extraoral and intraoral structures. Because many individuals have variations of normal oral anatomy, clinicians should be familiar with them. The variations often present as distinct oral conditions, but they are not pathologic.

ACKNOWLEDGMENTS

Clinical images were obtained at the Department of Oral Medicine, School of Dental Medicine, University of Pennsylvania and Department of Oral Medicine, Sibar Institute of Dental Sciences, Guntur, India. Special thanks to Drs Chalatip Chompund Na Ayudhya (University of Pennsylvania) and Samatha Yalamanchili (Sibar Institute of Dental Sciences) for assistance with capturing the clinical images.

REFERENCES

1. Haber J, Strasser S, Lloyd M, et al. The oral-systemic connection in primary care. Nurse Pract 2009;34(3):43–8.
2. Joseph BK, Kullman L, Sharma PN. The oral-systemic disease connection: a retrospective study. Clin Oral Investig 2016;20(8):2267–73.
3. Pedersen A, Sorensen CE, Proctor GB, et al. Salivary functions in mastication, taste and textural perception, swallowing and initial digestion. Oral Dis 2018;24(8):1399–416.
4. Touger-Decker R, Mobley C, Academy of N, et al. Position of the Academy of Nutrition and Dietetics: oral health and nutrition. J Acad Nutr Diet 2013; 113(5):693–701.
5. Andreeva VA, Kesse-Guyot E, Galan P, et al. Adherence to National Dietary Guidelines in Association with Oral Health Impact on Quality of Life. Nutrients 2018;10(5) [pii:E527].
6. Solemdal K, Sandvik L, Willumsen T, et al. The impact of oral health on taste ability in acutely hospitalized elderly. PLoS One 2012;7(5):e36557.
7. Kalogirou EM, Tosios KI, Nikitakis NG, et al. Transient lingual papillitis: A retrospective study of 11 cases and review of the literature. J Clin Exp Dent 2017;9(1):e157–62.
8. Kornerup IM, Senye M, Peters E. Transient lingual papillitis. Quintessence Int 2016;47(10): 871–5.
9. Rizos M, Spyropoulos MN. Van der Woude syndrome: a review. Cardinal signs, epidemiology, associated features, differential diagnosis, expressivity, genetic counselling and treatment. Eur J Orthod 2004;26(1):17–24.
10. Schutte BC, Basart AM, Watanabe Y, et al. Microdeletions at chromosome bands 1q32-q41 as a cause of Van der Woude syndrome. Am J Med Genet 1999; 84(2):145–50.
11. Suzuki K, Tsuchihashi Y. New attempt of personal identification by means of lip print. J Indian Dent Assoc 1970;42(1):8–9.
12. Tsuchihashi Y. Studies on personal identification by means of lip prints. Forensic Sci 1974;3(3):233–48.
13. Coward RC. The stability of lip pattern characteristics over time. J Forensic Odontostomatol 2007; 25(2):40–56.
14. Madani FM, Kuperstein AS. Normal variations of oral anatomy and common oral soft tissue lesions: evaluation and management. Med Clin North Am 2014; 98(6):1281–98.
15. Gorsky M, Buchner A, Fundoianu-Dayan D, et al. Fordyce's granules in the oral mucosa of adult Israeli Jews. Community Dent Oral Epidemiol 1986;14(4): 231–2.
16. Jha AK, Zeeshan MD, Jha Amar AK. Mucoscopy in lingual varicosities. Dermatol Pract Concept 2018; 8(1):54–5.
17. Muller S. Frictional Keratosis, Contact Keratosis and Smokeless Tobacco Keratosis: Features of Reactive White Lesions of the Oral Mucosa. Head Neck Pathol 2019;13(1):16–24.
18. Varoni E, Decani S. Images in clinical medicine. Geographic Tongue. N Engl J Med 2016;374(7):670.
19. Jacob CN, John TM, R J. Geographic tongue. Cleve Clin J Med 2016;83(8):565–6.

20. Damm DD, Fantasia JE. Bilateral white lesions of buccal mucosa. Morsicatio buccarum. Gen Dent 2006;54(6):442, 444.

21. Canaan TJ, Meehan SC. Variations of structure and appearance of the oral mucosa. Dent Clin North Am 2005;49(1):1–14, vii.

22. Walsh J, Tunkel D. Diagnosis and Treatment of Ankyloglossia in Newborns and Infants: A Review. JAMA Otolaryngol Head Neck Surg 2017;143(10): 1032–9.

23. Bakshi SS. Fissured tongue. Cleve Clin J Med 2019; 86(11):714.

Common Dental and Periodontal Diseases

Joel M. Laudenbach, DMD[a],*, Satish S. Kumar, DMD, MDSc, MS[b]

KEYWORDS

- Dental caries • Periapical abscess • Gingivitis • Periodontitis • Periodontal abscess • Pericoronitis
- Periimplant mucositis and periimplantitis

KEY POINTS

- Dental caries is a complex, multifactorial disease process triggered by bacterial biofilms in the presence of carbohydrates and acidic environment leading to loss of tooth structure.
- Addressing risk factors of caries development and early detection and management of carious lesions are critical in reducing the serious consequences of advanced caries, such as abscesses and tooth loss.
- Periodontal diseases include several diseases ranging from periodontitis to neoplasms affecting the periodontium (gingiva, periodontal ligament, cementum, and alveolar bone).
- Periodontitis is a complex, multifactorial, inflammatory disease caused by dysbiosis between bacterial biofilms and host inflammatory response. It is influenced by genetic factors, systemic diseases, and environmental factors, such as smoking.
- Periimplant diseases are inflammatory processes affecting the periimplant tissues; namely, periimplant mucositis and periimplantitis. Although periimplant mucositis affects the soft tissue component around the implant and is reversible by prompt treatment, periimplantitis causes destruction of underlying alveolar bone and is not reversible.

INTRODUCTION

Oral health is defined as "multi-faceted and includes the ability to speak, smile, taste, touch, chew, swallow and convey a range of emotions through facial expressions with confidence and without pain, discomfort and disease of the craniofacial complex."[1]

As the definition implies, oral diseases, such as dental caries, periodontal diseases, and eventual tooth loss that negatively affect oral health, ultimately affect the overall well-being of the individual in multidimensional facets, including the psychosocial aspects. Physicians, specialists, and allied health professionals hence become an integral part of managing and maintaining oral health of their patients along with dental professionals. Medical professionals can help with the oral health of their patients in various ways, such as screening for risk factors during medical history taking and educating their patients about the importance of oral health. Including oral health care providers as part of the referral network and following up with patients is crucial. Visual examination of the entire oral cavity, teeth, and gingiva (ie, gums) for caries, abscess, and periodontal inflammation to detect disease is a key part of any physical examination, especially during wellness visits. Certain preventive treatments, such as application of fluoride varnish and silver diamine fluoride, is being performed by physicians.[2,3] Advocating for oral health as physicians and understanding the serious implications of oral diseases serves the cause for better overall health.[4,5]

[a] Carolinas Center for Oral Health - Atrium Health, 1601 Abbey Place, Suite 220, Charlotte, NC 28209, USA;
[b] Arizona School of Dentistry and Oral Health, 5855 East Still Circle, Mesa, AZ 85206, USA
* Corresponding author.
E-mail address: Joel.Laudenbach@atriumhealth.org

Dermatol Clin 38 (2020) 413–420
https://doi.org/10.1016/j.det.2020.05.002

ORAL DISEASES

Oral diseases, in particular dental caries and periodontal diseases, affect about 3.5 billion people around the globe and are among the most common preventable and noncommunicable infectious diseases.[6] Despite significant progress in oral health care, the burden of oral disease remains, especially in low socioeconomic populations with limited access to care.[7] The quality of life of patients afflicted with severe oral diseases is very poor. This article focuses on common oral diseases and conditions that physicians and their affiliates are likely to encounter in their medical practices, including dental caries, dental abscess, dental erosion, dental attrition, gingivitis, periodontitis, necrotizing gingivitis, necrotizing periodontitis, and periimplant diseases that affect dental implants. Recognition and management of these not only aids in improving oral health but also the overall health and well-being of patients.

DENTAL CARIES

Dental caries is considered the most common disease in the world.[3] It affects about 2.3 billion adults and 530 million children worldwide.[3] "Dental caries is a biofilm-mediated, diet-modulated, multifactorial, noncommunicable, dynamic disease resulting in net mineral loss of dental hard tissues. It is determined by biological, behavioral, psychosocial, and environmental factors. As a consequence of this process, a caries or carious lesion develops on dental hard tissues."[8] The biofilm refers to the complex environment composed of microorganisms and their extracellular matrix. There are about 800 species of bacteria in the oral cavity. The acidic pH environment mediated by this biofilm enriched by carbohydrates leads to the net mineral loss (demineralization) of tooth surface. Frequent intake of sugars and an acidic environment shifts the delicate symbiosis between oral commensal microorganisms to a state of dysbiosis with growth of bacteria such as *Streptococcus mutans* and *Lactobacillus* species.[9] When present clinically, caries is referred to as carious lesions. They affect both primary and permanent teeth and can be present on the crown (coronal) portion of the tooth in various surfaces, such as the occluding surfaces (occlusal), interproximal surfaces (mesial and distal), cheek-facing or lip-facing surfaces (facial/buccal) and tongue-facing (lingual) surfaces, and/or root portion of the tooth. They can cause a cavity (cavitated lesion) or may be present without causing a visible cavity (noncavitated lesion). Caries can penetrate through the layers of teeth: enamel, followed by dentin, and to the pulp[10]

(**Fig. 1**). Childhood caries and caries affecting geriatric patients have slightly different risk factors. For example, children are typically prone to excessive exposure to refined sugars through their diets and also inadequate plaque control. Older adults can have physical restrictions, in addition to taking multiple medications, which may cause dry mouth and hyposalivation. Cognitive deficits caused by dementia, Alzheimer disease, functional deficits caused by stroke, and lack of social support and access to care are all contributing factors to rapid oral health deterioration among older adults.[11]

Management of dental caries involves risk identification and mitigation, nonrestorative treatments, and restorative treatments. Age-appropriate dietary counseling to reduce intake

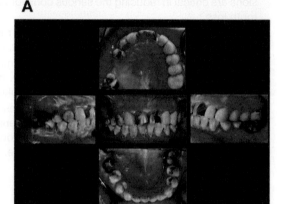

A

B

Fig. 1. (A) A full-mouth series of photographs showing extensive dental caries. Caries destruction is noted in all surfaces (occlusal, incisal, and cervical regions) of many teeth. (B) Full-mouth series of radiographs of the same patient shown in Fig. 1B. Caries involvement in various stages can be appreciated here. For example, lower right first molar and lower left second molar show complete loss of crown to caries and have developed periapical lesion, possibly a granuloma (*stars*).

of food and drinks containing high sugar levels aids in reducing the incidence of caries.[12] Nonrestorative treatment of cavitated lesions in primary and permanent teeth is recommended to be performed with 38% silver diamine fluoride solution. Silver diamine fluoride is an alkaline solution of silver and fluoride shown to be effective in arresting coronal caries in primary dentition and also root caries in older adults.[13] For noncavitated lesions, based on the surface of the tooth affected by caries (occlusal, approximal, facial or lingual, and root surface), different treatment options are recommended. Examples of these nonrestorative treatment options include sealants, 5% sodium fluoride (NaF) varnish, 1.23% acidulated phosphate fluoride gel, resin infiltration, and 0.2% NaF mouthrinse.[14] Restorative treatments provided by dentists include use of different restorative materials, including amalgams, resins, and cements.

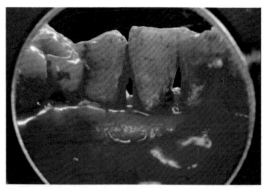

Fig. 2. A close-up of dental plaque biofilm and calculus on teeth surfaces. These buildups are hard concretions formed over months, and are difficult to remove by routine toothbrushing. Removal (ie, scaling) by trained professionals using specialized dental instruments is needed.

PERIAPICAL ABSCESS

Untreated dental caries can lead to abscess formation, typically in the periapical region. Abscesses may remain local but, if left untreated, can spread to adjacent tissues causing space infections, fever, swelling, lymphadenopathy, trismus, and even distant spreading, which may potentially become life-threatening. Expedient diagnosis and treatment are warranted to mitigate the consequences of periapical abscess. Treatment ranges from root canal therapy to extraction of the offending tooth. Systemic antibiotics may be necessary in certain situations, especially with systemic involvement, to control the spread of infection.[15] In large abscesses, incision and drainage of the abscess is necessary, along with antibiotics, until definitive treatment, such as extraction, is completed.

GINGIVITIS

Periodontium is a collective term that refers to the surrounding structures of a tooth. It comprises the gingiva, periodontal ligament, cementum, and alveolar bone.[16] Periodontal diseases affect about 800 million people worldwide, with about 270 million people having edentulism and severe tooth loss.[3] A plethora of causal factors and systemic diseases cause periodontal disease, ranging from microbial biofilms to genetic syndromes and malignancies.[17,18]

Gingivitis refers to the inflammation of gingiva, usually in response to plaque biofilm accumulation (**Fig. 2**).[19] Gingivitis can also result in the absence of plaque biofilm from several causes, ranging from genetic and developmental disorders, infections (bacterial, viral, fungal), autoimmune diseases, to neoplasms. These causes are uncommon and are not discussed here. Gingivitis caused by dental plaque biofilm is defined as "an inflammatory lesion resulting from interactions between the dental plaque biofilm and the host's immune-inflammatory response, which remains contained within the gingiva and does not extend to the periodontal attachment (cementum, periodontal ligament and alveolar bone). Such inflammation remains confined to the gingiva and does not extend beyond the mucogingival junction and is reversible by reducing levels of dental plaque at and apical to the gingival margin."[20,21] As the definition states, gingivitis is confined to the gingiva and does not affect deeper structures of the periodontium. It is usually reversible once the cause is identified and treated.

Dental plaque biofilm is a complex mixture of microorganisms and their substrates. Biofilm elicits a host inflammatory response, and gingivitis manifests only when there is an imbalance between the biofilm presence and the inflammatory response specific to the host, a process referred to as dysbiosis.[22] Gingivitis severity can be modified by several other factors, such as smoking, diabetes, nutritional factors, certain prescription drugs, sex hormones, and hematological conditions. When additional factors are contributing to the severity of gingivitis in addition to plaque biofilm, these additional factors need to be controlled to treat gingivitis. Some of the classic signs of inflammation are usually present in patients with gingivitis: redness (erythema), swelling (edema), and pain (soreness). Clinically, erythema or redness of the gingival margin is noted with bleeding when provoked during routine brushing or during clinical examination using a periodontal probe. Patients are likely to report bleeding gums, bad breath, and pain. They may also complain about difficulty with chewing and eating if the pain and discomfort are severe. Treatment usually involves physical removal of local factors, such as plaque and calculus, by a dentist or a dental hygienist, a process referred to as scaling. The patients usually receive oral hygiene instructions that include proper brushing techniques, interproximal (between teeth) cleaning techniques using floss or interproximal brushes, and use of mouth rinse.[23] Oral hygiene maintenance by patients at home is crucial for prevention of recurrence of gingivitis. Underlying modifying factors, such as smoking or diabetes, should ideally be controlled for long-term management. Any tooth-related factors, such as a fractured tooth or restoration acting as a plaque trap, require correction as well.[24] Prevention is the best way to manage gingivitis caused by plaque accumulation. Brushing twice daily and flossing, along with the use of antibacterial mouth rinse diligently, ensures regular removal of plaque biofilm around gingival margins on the tooth surfaces.[25]

PERIODONTITIS

When gingival inflammation progresses to cause further damage of the underlying connective tissue and alveolar bone surrounding the tooth, it is referred to as periodontitis. Periodontitis is also an inflammatory condition mediated by dysbiosis, the imbalance between microbial biofilms and host inflammatory response. Periodontitis is influenced by genetic factors, environmental factors such as smoking, and systemic diseases such as diabetes. There are several systemic diseases that can directly cause periodontal attachment loss in the absence of local factors. They are rare, and readers are directed to other publications for details.[8]

Two major forms of periodontitis were identified previously as chronic and aggressive periodontitis. Recently, these 2 forms of periodontitis were shown to be not different from a pathophysiologic perspective.[26] Periodontitis is currently categorized into different stages (stages I–IV) and grades (grades A–C) based on severity of disease, measured by different clinical parameters, such as bone loss and the rate of progression respectively.[27] Stage I disease is considered a mild form of disease, stage II is moderate, stage III is severe, and stage IV is an advanced form of disease where the patient is likely to become edentulous, losing the entire dentition. A slowly progressing periodontitis is graded A, whereas moderately progressing disease is considered grade B, followed by the rapidly progressing form of disease being grade C.[27]

Clinically, most patients present with local factors, such as calculus, inflamed gingival tissues that may bleed on brushing, deeper periodontal pockets, mobility of teeth, and/or discomfort on chewing (**Figs. 3** and **4**). The characteristic that makes periodontitis difficult to detect early is the lack of pain associated with the destruction of connective tissue and alveolar bone. Hence, most patients seek care late into the disease progression if they are not routinely undergoing dental evaluation.

Treatment of periodontitis typically involves nonsurgical forms of treatment: scaling and root planing using specialized instruments and use of ultrasonic and piezoelectric scalers. Short-term courses of systemic antibiotics and topical antiseptics, such as chlorhexidine 0.12% mouth rinse, are prescribed by the treating dentist or periodontist on an individualized basis to aid in control of bacterial biofilms and mitigate further inflammatory destruction. Diligent oral care at home by the patient is essential for the success of periodontal therapy.[28] Any residual periodontal pockets or advanced disease status that has not improved with nonsurgical therapy will undergo surgical periodontal therapy, where removal of local factors, resulting in reduction of inflammation, is accomplished by gingival flap elevation. Advances have been made to achieve periodontal regeneration with biologics and bone grafts in certain conducive periodontal osseous defects.

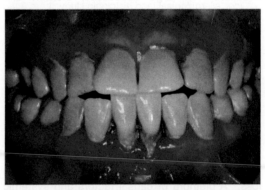

Fig. 3. Tissue response to local factors. The mandibular lower central incisors have gross calculus. Note the gingival tissue response to the calculus buildup: erythema, bleeding, edema, and recession indicating loss of alveolar bone in the facial aspect. Note also the early signs of gingivitis on maxillary central and lateral incisors to low presence of plaque biofilm and calculus.

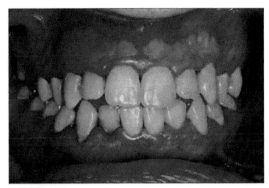

Fig. 4. This patient presented with generalized gingival inflammation in response to supragingival and subgingival calculus. The gingival margin in general is edematous, shiny, and bleeds easily. Note the presence of subgingival calculus (under the gingival sulcus) barely showing clinically. Note also the gingival inflammation and early abscess formation between the apical region of maxillary right canine and lateral incisor region.

Periodontitis is a chronic disease and goes through periods of exacerbation in susceptible individuals. Hence, periodontal maintenance tailored to each patient's needs is recommended for patients with periodontitis where ongoing vigilance and the needed treatment of recurrent disease can be accomplished before advanced destruction ensues.[29]

PERIODONTAL ABSCESS

On occasion, periodontal disease can manifest in the form of an abscess localized to the affected tooth (**Fig. 5**) or as multiple abscesses affecting many teeth (**Fig. 6**).[30] Clinical signs and symptoms are similar to periapical abscess, except that purulence is typically noted as an exudate from the gingival sulcus. Sinus tracts and fistulae formation can be noted when periodontal abscess gets large and when multiple teeth are affected.

PERICORONITIS

Another common diagnosis is acute pain associated with gingival tissues surrounding erupting or impacted third molars (ie, wisdom teeth). The gingival tissues surrounding these teeth may become inflamed because of food impaction and/or dental caries involving these teeth. This condition can progress to an acute infection and potentially spread to surrounding fascial spaces with associated complications, such as trismus and airway compromise. Localized pain without evidence of infection may be managed with analgesics and local debridement performed by a

A

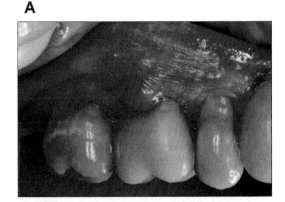

B

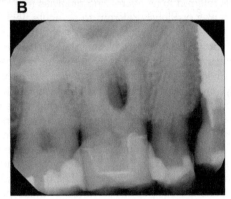

Fig. 5. (*A*) A well-defined marginal gingival swelling that expressed purulence on gentle palpation. The periodontal probe measured more than 10 mm in the midbuccal area, indicating severe bone loss in the furcation area. A healthy gingival sulcus (pocket) is equal to or less than 3 mm. (*B*) A periapical radiograph shows the severe bone loss in the furcation region of the tooth, confirming the clinical finding of deep periodontal probing, and also the reason for the appearance of a periodontal abscess.

dentist. Infection associated with this condition may be managed with antibiotics and antiseptic rinses, such as chlorhexidine 0.12%. In these cases, referral to a dentist is required for definitive

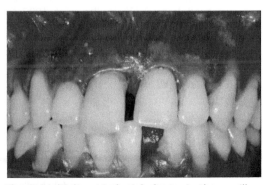

Fig. 6. Multiple periodontal abscess in the maxillary arch in an uncontrolled diabetic patient.

management, such as potential extraction of the causative tooth.[31]

NECROTIZING PERIODONTAL DISEASES (ACUTE NECROTIZING ULCERATIVE GINGIVITIS AND PERIODONTITIS)

Necrotizing periodontal diseases are unique periodontal diseases and are rare compared with ubiquitous plaque-induced gingivitis and periodontitis. Spirochetes in an immunocompromised situation cause a rapid, painful necrosis of gingival tissues that must be treated quickly. When the necrosis affects only the gingival tissues, the condition is referred to as necrotizing gingivitis (**Fig. 7**), which was previously referred to as acute necrotizing ulcerative gingivitis and, when the destruction progresses to involve the underlying connective tissue and alveolar bone, it is referred to as necrotizing periodontitis, which was previously referred to as acute necrotizing ulcerative periodontitis. Clinically, unlike periodontitis associated with plaque and calculus as discussed previously, patients report severe pain and discomfort and their symptoms are typically acute, having started a few days or weeks previously. A thin, white, keratotic film on an inflamed gingival tissue with punched-out papillae is noted in these patients. Halitosis is profound in some patients, with difficulty in opening the mouth, talking, and chewing. Treatment involves prescription of antibiotics, such as metronidazole, along with local debridement of local factors and gentle cleansing of necrotic tissue. Topical antiseptics, such as chlorhexidine 0.12% mouth rinse, are helpful.

PERIIMPLANT DISEASES

With the advent of dental implants to replace missing teeth, the prevalence continues to increase significantly. According to a recent study based on US National Health and Nutrition Examination Surveys (NHANES) data, the prevalence has increased from 0.7% in the year 1999 to 2000 to 5.7% in the year 2015 to 2016 and is projected to increase to 23% in the year 2026.[32] Dysbiotic state triggered by plaque biofilms and host immune system causing periodontal diseases around natural teeth also affects dental implants. The anatomic difference between natural teeth and dental implants in function makes onset and progress of periimplant diseases quicker than with natural teeth. Natural teeth are surrounded by complex and structurally sound connective tissue and periodontal ligament fibers compared with dental implants. When bacterial biofilms accumulate around dental implants, inflammation

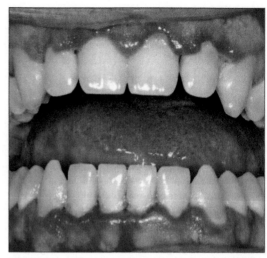

Fig. 7. Necrotizing gingivitis in a 22-year old male patient. Note the characteristic necrosis of gingival tissues and also the punched-out papillae between maxillary right central and lateral incisors, maxillary left central and lateral incisors, lateral incisor and canine.

ensues around the gingival tissues, resulting in erythema, edema, and bleeding. When the inflammation is restricted to soft tissues, it is referred to as periimplant mucositis.[33–35] As soon as the mucosal inflammation progresses to destruction of alveolar bone, it is referred to as periimplantitis.[36] History of periodontal disease, lack of good oral health maintenance,[37] certain systemic diseases (eg, uncontrolled diabetes), medications (eg, bisphosphonates, selective serotonin reuptake inhibitors), and history of radiotherapy have been shown to contribute to periimplant disease leading to implant failures.[38] Clinically, besides

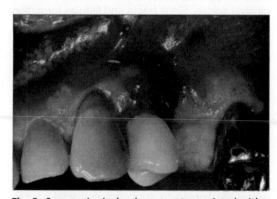

Fig. 8. Severe gingival enlargement associated with a failing implant in maxillary left first premolar region. Purulence and bleeding were expressed on gentle palpation. Radiograph showed severe bone loss confirming the diagnosis of periimplantitis.

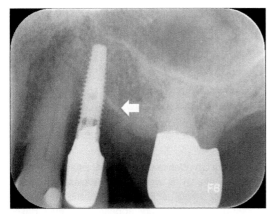

Fig. 9. Periapical radiograph of implant in **Fig. 8** showing extensive bone loss around the implant (*arrow*).

erythema and bleeding, occasional purulence is noted along the sulcus of the dental implant sites (**Figs. 8** and **9**). Hence, maintenance of dental implants with effective home care oral hygiene as well routine dental visits is crucial for long-term success of dental implants. Prevention of periimplant diseases is preferred to treatment because treatment of ailing implants is challenging and unpredictable. Treatment involves both nonsurgical debridement of implant surface along with topical antiseptics and systemic antibiotics as needed. Surgical therapy is indicated with bone loss and is conducive to bone grafting. When an implant has lost most of its supporting bone, reducing its functional capacity, or the implant becomes mobile, it is considered untreatable and requires removal. Hence, clinicians must stress the importance of maintaining good health around dental implants, similar to natural teeth.

SUMMARY

This article provides a brief overview of common dental and periodontal conditions ranging from dental caries to periodontal and periimplant diseases. Early detection of these conditions and appropriate management, including prompt referral to dental professionals, is critical to avoid further complications.

DISCLOSURE

The authors have nothing to disclose.

REFERENCES

1. Glick M, Williams DM, Kleinman DV, et al. A new definition for oral health developed by the FDI World Dental Federation opens the door to a universal definition of oral health. J Am Dent Assoc 2016; 147(12):915–7.
2. Sudhanthar S, Lapinski J, Turner J, et al. Improving oral health through dental fluoride varnish application in a primary care paediatric practice. BMJ Open Qual 2019;8(2):e000589.
3. Bernstein RS, Johnston B, Mackay K, et al. Implementation of a primary care physician-led Cavity Clinic using silver diamine fluoride. J Public Health Dent 2019;79(3):193–7.
4. Watt RG, Daly B, Allison P, et al. Ending the neglect of global oral health: time for radical action. Lancet 2019;394(10194):261–72.
5. Fisher-Owens SA. The interprofessional role in dental caries management: ways medical providers can support oral health (perspectives from a physician). Dent Clin North Am 2019;63(4):669–77.
6. GBD 2017 Disease and Injury Incidence and Prevalence Collaborators. Global, regional, and national incidence, prevalence, and years lived with disability for 354 diseases and injuries for 195 countries and territories, 1990-2017: a systematic analysis for the Global Burden of Disease Study 2017. Lancet 2019;393(10190):e44 [Erratum appears in Lancet 2019;393(10190):e44].
7. Peres MA, Macpherson LMD, Weyant RJ, et al. Oral diseases: a global public health challenge. Lancet 2019;394(10194):249–60 [Erratum appears in Lancet 2019;394(10203):1010].
8. Pitts NB, Zero DT, Marsh PD, et al. Dental caries. Nat Rev Dis Primers 2017;3:17030.
9. Nascimento MM. Approaches to Modulate Biofilm Ecology. Dent Clin North Am 2019;63(4):581–94.
10. Machiulskiene V, Campus G, Carvalho JC, et al. Terminology of dental caries and dental caries management: consensus report of a workshop organized by ORCA and cariology research group of IADR. Caries Res 2020;54(1):7–14.
11. Marchini L, Ettinger R, Hartshorn J. Personalized dental caries management for frail older adults and persons with special needs. Dent Clin North Am 2019;63(4):631–51.
12. Marshall TA. Dietary implications for dental caries: a practical approach on dietary counseling. Dent Clin North Am 2019;63(4):595–605.
13. Seifo N, Cassie H, Radford JR, et al. Silver diamine fluoride for managing carious lesions: an umbrella review. BMC Oral Health 2019;19(1):145.
14. Slayton RL, Urquhart O, Araujo MWB, et al. Evidence-based clinical practice guideline on nonrestorative treatments for carious lesions: A report from the American Dental Association. J Am Dent Assoc 2018;149(10):837–49.e19.
15. Lockhart PB, Tampi MP, Abt E, et al. Evidence-based clinical practice guideline on antibiotic use for the urgent management of pulpal- and periapical-related dental pain and intraoral swelling:

A report from the American Dental Association. J Am Dent Assoc 2019;150(11):906–21.e12.

16. Lang NP, Bartold PM. Periodontal health. J Periodontol 2018;89(Suppl 1):S9–16.

17. Papapanou PN, Sanz M, Buduneli N, et al. Periodontitis: consensus report of workgroup 2 of the 2017 World Workshop on the Classification of Periodontal and Peri-Implant Diseases and Conditions. J Periodontol 2018;89(Suppl 1):S173–82.

18. Jepsen S, Caton JG, Albandar JM, et al. Periodontal manifestations of systemic diseases and developmental and acquired conditions: Consensus report of workgroup 3 of the 2017 World Workshop on the Classification of Periodontal and Peri-Implant Diseases and Conditions. J Periodontol 2018;89(Suppl 1):S237–48.

19. Murakami S, Mealey BL, Mariotti A, et al. Dental plaque-induced gingival conditions. J Periodontol 2018;89(Suppl 1):S17–27.

20. Trombelli L, Farina R, Silva CO, et al. Plaque-induced gingivitis: Case definition and diagnostic considerations. J Periodontol 2018;89(Suppl 1):S46–73.

21. Chapple ILC, Mealey BL, Van Dyke TE, et al. Periodontal health and gingival diseases and conditions on an intact and a reduced periodontium: Consensus report of workgroup 1 of the 2017 World Workshop on the Classification of Periodontal and Peri-Implant Diseases and Conditions. J Periodontol 2018;89(Suppl 1):S74–84.

22. Hajishengallis G, Lamont RJ. Beyond the red complex and into more complexity: the polymicrobial synergy and dysbiosis (PSD) model of periodontal disease etiology. Mol Oral Microbiol 2012;27(6):409–19.

23. Worthington HV, MacDonald L, Poklepovic Pericic T, et al. Home use of interdental cleaning devices, in addition to toothbrushing, for preventing and controlling periodontal diseases and dental caries. Cochrane Database Syst Rev 2019;(4):CD012018.

24. Ercoli C, Caton JG. Dental prostheses and tooth-related factors. J Periodontol 2018;89(Suppl 1):S223–36.

25. Chapple IL, Van der Weijden F, Doerfer C, et al. Primary prevention of periodontitis: managing gingivitis. J Clin Periodontol 2015;42(Suppl 16):S71–6.

26. Fine DH, Patil AG, Loos BG. Classification and diagnosis of aggressive periodontitis. J Periodontol 2018;89(Suppl 1):S103–19.

27. Tonetti MS, Greenwell H, Kornman KS. Staging and grading of periodontitis: Framework and proposal of a new classification and case definition. J Periodontol 2018;89(Suppl 1):S159–72 [Erratum appears in J Periodontol 2018;89(12):1475].

28. Smiley CJ, Tracy SL, Abt E, et al. Evidence-based clinical practice guideline on the nonsurgical treatment of chronic periodontitis by means of scaling and root planing with or without adjuncts. J Am Dent Assoc 2015;146(7):525–35.

29. Farooqi OA, Wehler CJ, Gibson G, et al. Appropriate recall interval for periodontal maintenance: a systematic review. J Evid Based Dent Pract 2015;15(4):171–81 [Erratum appears in J Evid Based Dent Pract 2016;16(1):79].

30. Herrera D, Alonso B, de Arriba L, et al. Acute periodontal lesions. Periodontol 2000 2014;65(1):149–77.

31. Renton T, Wilson NH. Problems with erupting wisdom teeth: signs, symptoms, and management. Br J Gen Pract 2016;66(649):e606–8.

32. Elani HW, Starr JR, Da Silva JD, et al. Trends in dental implant use in the U.S., 1999-2016, and projections to 2026. J Dent Res 2018;97(13):1424–30.

33. Renvert S, Persson GR, Pirih FQ, et al. Peri-implant health, peri-implant mucositis, and peri-implantitis: Case definitions and diagnostic considerations. J Periodontol 2018;89(Suppl 1):S304–12.

34. Heitz-Mayfield LJA, Salvi GE. Peri-implant mucositis. J Periodontol 2018;89(Suppl 1):S257–66.

35. Berglundh T, Armitage G, Araujo MG, et al. Peri-implant diseases and conditions: consensus report of workgroup 4 of the 2017 world workshop on the classification of periodontal and peri-implant diseases and conditions. J Periodontol 2018;89(Suppl 1):S313–8.

36. Schwarz F, Derks J, Monje A, et al. Peri-implantitis. J Periodontol 2018;89(Suppl 1):S267–90.

37. Atieh MA, Pang JK, Lian K, et al. Predicting peri-implant disease: Chi-square automatic interaction detection (CHAID) decision tree analysis of risk indicators. J Periodontol 2019;90(8):834–46.

38. Kumar PS. Systemic risk factors for the development of periimplant diseases. Implant Dent 2019;28(2):115–9.

Oral Biopsy Techniques

Rabie M. Shanti, DMD, MD[a,*], Takako Tanaka, DDS, FDS, RCSEd[b],
David C. Stanton, DMD, MD[c,d,e]

KEYWORDS

• Oral biopsy • Lip biopsy • Oral cancer • Oral dysplasia • Leukoplakia

KEY POINTS

- Scalpel or punch biopsy are recommended techniques for the biopsy of oral lesions.
- Excisional biopsy should be avoided if malignancy is of concern, and should be reserved for lesions where excisional biopsy is likely to be definitive.
- Obtaining two specimens for hematoxylin-eosin and direct immunofluorescence (DIF) is imperative if autoimmune blistering disease (AIBD) is of concern.
- Oral biopsies are safely performed in the outpatient setting in most patients with careful attention to local anatomy and adequate local anesthesia.

INTRODUCTION

The oral cavity is the gateway to the body, serving as the portal of entry for the foods and the liquids we consume, and most microorganisms and medications we are exposed to and all the chemical and physical irritants that may be associated with them. Furthermore, in select patients, the oral cavity mucosa is exposed to tobacco products and/or alcohol, which are known risk factors for oral cancer, and various dental materials and oral hygiene products. The oral cavity houses a myriad of tissue types (eg, teeth, minor salivary glands, taste buds) with varying embryologic origins and physiologic functions that are intimately associated with one another. As a result, the mucosa of the oral cavity is susceptible to the development of reactive, inflammatory, infectious, immune-related, and neoplastic conditions (**Fig. 1**), and as within any anatomic region afflicted with disease, proper patient management starts with establishing the correct diagnosis. Therefore, biopsy of a soft tissue lesion is a critical diagnostic

tool to aid histologic diagnosis; however, its clinical relevance depends on a sound clinicopathologic assessment of the patient's condition. In this article we review the armamentarium and technical considerations involved with performing a biopsy of a soft tissue lesion of the oral cavity.

LOCAL ANESTHESIA

As with any surgical procedure, profound anesthesia is imperative to properly perform the procedure, and delivery of a local anesthetic near a terminal nerve branch of the trigeminal nerve (the fifth cranial nerve) is required for oral biopsy. Local anesthesia is delivered either as an infiltration (delivery of local anesthetic around the periphery of the lesion) or through a nerve block technique (**Fig. 2**). The benefits and disadvantages of local anesthetic filtration technique for oral mucosal biopsy are listed in **Box 1**. Therefore, it is critical when using a local infiltration technique to avoid injecting directly into the lesion. For most oral lesions requiring biopsy, adequate anesthesia is

a Department of Otorhinolaryngology/Head and Neck Surgery, University of Pennsylvania Health System, 3400 Civic Center Boulevard, 4th Floor, South Pavilion, Philadelphia, PA 19104, USA; b Department of Oral Medicine, School of Dental Medicine, University of Pennsylvania, 240 South 40th Street, Philadelphia, PA 19104, USA; c Oral & Maxillofacial Surgery, University of Pennsylvania Health System, Philadelphia, PA, USA; d Oral & Maxillofacial Surgery, Children's Hospital of Philadelphia, Philadelphia, PA, USA; e Department of Oral & Maxillofacial Surgery, Perelman Center, 4th Floor, South Pavilion, 3400 Civic Center Boulevard, Philadelphia, PA 19104, USA
* Corresponding author.
E-mail address: rabie.shanti@pennmedicine.upenn.edu

Dermatol Clin 38 (2020) 421–427
https://doi.org/10.1016/j.det.2020.05.003

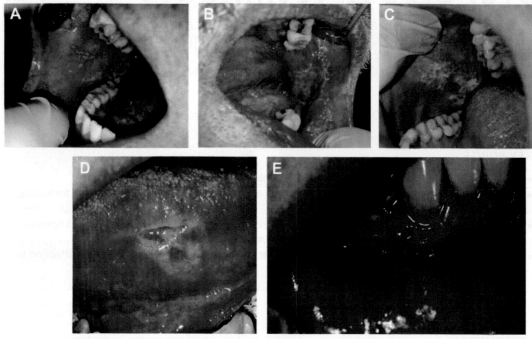

Fig. 1. (*A*) Oral lichen planus (reticular type). (*B*) Erosive lichen planus. (*C*) Leukoplakia. (*D*) Syphilitic chancre of the tongue. (*E*) Subepithelial fluid-filled bullae in a patient with mucous membrane pemphigoid. ([E] *Courtesy of* E Ko, DDS, Philadelphia, PA.)

achieved with local infiltration technique without the need for a block. Furthermore, in the absence of a medical contraindication or history of drug allergy/sensitivity/reaction to vasoconstrictor (ie, epinephrine), the use of a vasoconstrictor allows for better hemostasis and longer duration of the anesthesia. Of note, irrespective of local

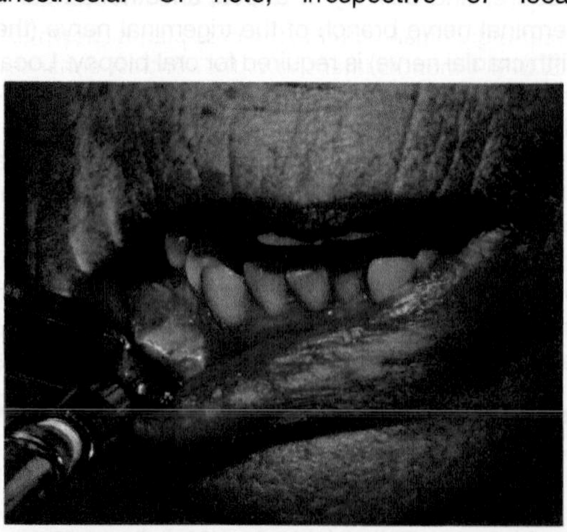

Fig. 2. Right mental nerve block in preparation for biopsy of right lower lip lesion. To achieve a block of the mental nerve, local anesthetic is injected along the area of the mental foramen, which is palpable in most patients. If the mental foramen is not palpable then the local anesthetic is deposited deep to the mucosa in the region between the two premolar teeth.

anesthetic delivery technique, it is critical to always aspirate before injection to avoid intravascular delivery of local anesthetic and vasoconstrictor. Furthermore, to optimize patient comfort during the biopsy procedure, we recommend the use of a topical anesthetic (ie, 20% benzocaine) for 1 minute using a cotton swab before mucosal perforation with the needle, and deposition of the local anesthetic solution over 1 to 2 minutes.

BIOPSY TECHNIQUES

Oral biopsies are either incisional or excisional. Several biopsy techniques have been described for skin lesions, such as scalpel, shave, punch, scoop (saucerization), curettage, and scissor technique.[1] Within the oral cavity proper, the scalpel and punch biopsy techniques are recommended. In select cases, brush cytology is considered.[2,3] Incisional biopsies usually are performed with a punch biopsy (3–4 mm) (**Fig. 3**) or scalpel, whereas excisional biopsies are commonly performed with a scalpel (our preference is for the use of a #15 stainless steel scalpel blade) (**Fig. 4**). Incisional biopsy technique is recommended for the biopsy of large lesions (**Fig. 5**) and lesions that are suspicious for malignancy. In cases of suspected malignancy, preservation of the borders of the lesions is the borders of the lesions allows the extirpative surgeon to maximize the ability to achieve an R0 resection (surgical extirpation with microscopically margin-negative resection). Orosco and colleagues[4] published an extensive analysis of the positive surgical margins in the 10 most common solid cancers using the National Cancer Data Base and identified oral cancer as the most common cancer with the highest positive surgical margin rate in women and men combined. Being able to achieve an R0 resection is complicated when the biopsy removes all clinically visible portions of the lesion. Nonetheless, with certain small lesions, it is impossible to perform an incisional biopsy and in this situation, an excisional biopsy is unavoidable. Therefore, in such a situation when a malignancy is suspected with a small lesion that is not amenable to an incisional biopsy, referral to the cancer surgeon who will provide definitive treatment or biopsy of the lesion with photograph documentation to orient the extirpative surgeon is our recommendation. Excisional biopsy should only be considered based on the physician's clinical expertise that excision of the

important for proper oncologic extirpation. The importance of this cannot be overstated. As with resection of any malignancy, achieving negative surgical margins is the goal and ability to visualize

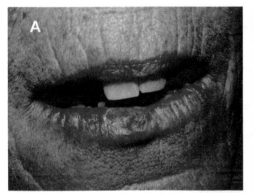
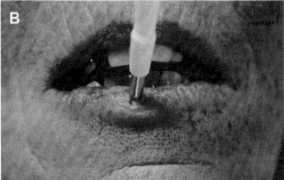
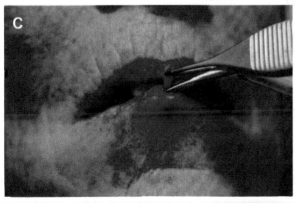
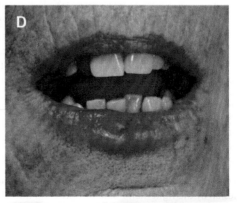

Fig. 3. (A) Ulcerative lesion of the right lower lip with final diagnosis of squamous cell carcinoma. (B) Use of 3 mm punch biopsy with firm twisting action to cut through lesion and deeper layers. (C) Use of scissors to amputate tissue specimen. (D) Reapproximation of tissue edges with use of 3-0 Vicryl (polyglactin 910) suture manufactured by Ethicon, Somerville, NJ, USA.

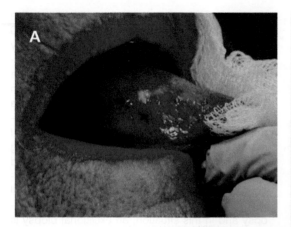
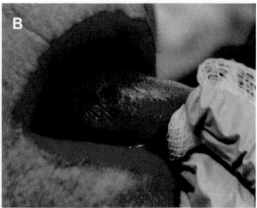
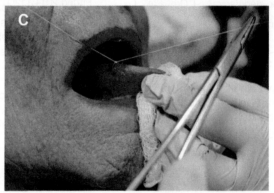

Fig. 4. (*A*) White, homogeneous, nonulcerated white lesion along the lateral border of the right tongue that does not wipe off. (*B*) Postbiopsy tongue defect following elliptical incision technique using #15 scalpel. (*C*) Reapproximation of tissue edges with use of 3–0 Vicryl (polyglactin 910) suture.

lesion is the appropriate definitive/curative treatment.

Following completion of tissue procurement during the biopsy procedure, reapproximation of

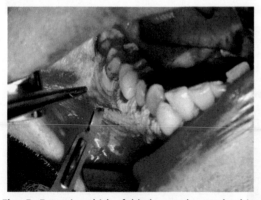

Fig. 5. Extensive thick, folded, nonulcerated white lesion of the right mandibular gingiva and buccal mucosa in a patient with proliferative verrucous leukoplakia undergoing incisional biopsy using #15 scalpel blade. Because of the size of the lesion excisional biopsy is not feasible.

the mucosa is achieved using either a permanent or an absorbable suture as feasible. It is our preference to use an absorbable suture either 3–0 or 4–0 Vicryl (polyglactin 910) suture (Ethicon, Johnson & Johnson, Sommerville, NJ) on a tapered point needle for mucosa because of the delicacy of mucosa.

SPECIAL CONSIDERATIONS
Oral Squamous Cell Carcinoma

Squamous cell carcinoma (SCC) makes up 90% of all oral cancers. The most significant negative prognosticator for oral SCC is the presence of cervical lymph node metastasis.[5,6] When cervical lymph node metastasis occurs, survival rate is reduced by 50% or more.[7] The incidence of cervical lymph node metastasis in patients with oral SCC is approximately 40%.[7] Therefore, staging and management of the cervical lymph nodes of the neck is a critical aspect of the management of oral SCC. The decision of when to perform a neck dissection (cervical lymphadenectomy) (**Fig. 6**) in a clinically negative neck evaluation

As with any surgical procedure, thorough understanding of anatomic structures in the region of the procedure is imperative as to not cause injury to critical structure (ie, ducts of salivary glands and nerves) and avoiding injury to vascular structures for risk of hematoma or hemorrhage. Appreciation of the local anatomy is an important consideration for any clinician embarking on any invasive procedure.

Autoimmune Blistering Diseases

The autoimmune blistering diseases (AIBDs) are a group of disorders affecting mucosa and skin, which include pemphigus, pemphigoid, IgA-mediated dermatoses, and epidermolysis bullosa acquista. It is not uncommon for the oral cavity to be the initial site of involvement, particularly in pemphigus vulgaris (PV) and mucous membrane pemphigoid (MMP).[10–12] Oral lesions can present as subtle, nonspecific erosive or/and ulcerative lesions rather than vesicles or bullae because the lesions are easily traumatized by eating, drinking, and/or various parafunctional habits. An early and accurate diagnosis of AIBD is critical because delayed treatment can eventually cause life-threatening complications.

It is imperative to obtain two specimens for hematoxylin-eosin and direct immunofluorescence (DIF) evaluation for diagnosing AIBD.[10–13] Although a specimen is stored in 10% formalin for routine hematoxylin-eosin, the DIF specimen needs to be stored in Michel transport medium to detect specific immunofluorescence staining depending on AIBD. The DIF specimens must be taken from perilesional (within 1 cm) or normal-appearing tissue.[13,14] Biopsy solely from the ulcerated or severely erosive lesion or "peeled" bed has no diagnostic value because the intraepithelial destruction (eg, PV) or subepithelial destruction

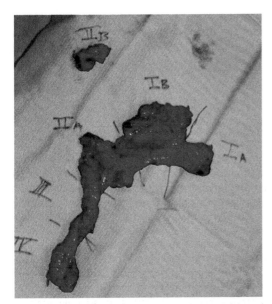

Fig. 6. Intraoperative photograph of cervical lymph node packet following completion of selective neck dissection of levels I-IV of the neck.

(cN0) has been widely investigated with the most reliable histologic predictor of cervical node metastasis in early stage oral SCC being depth of invasion.[8] Furthermore, 15% of patients with oral SCC with clinically and radiographically negative cervical lymph nodes that undergo a neck dissection or observation of their cervical lymph nodes go on to develop neck recurrence.[9] Therefore, to aid in ascertaining the depth of invasion in a lesion clinically suspicious for SCC, it is important to extend the depth of the biopsy deep to the mucosa (**Fig. 7**) for the pathologist to differentiate between invasive SCC and carcinoma in situ, and the pathologist being able to ascertain the depth of invasion.

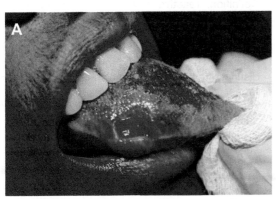
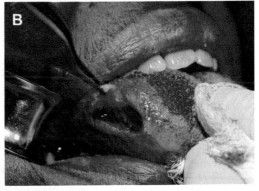

Fig. 7. (A) Endophytic, ulcerated lesion with rolled borders along the lateral border of the right oral tongue. (B) Incisional biopsy using #15 scalpel for biopsy of lesion. Note depth of biopsy to obtain a cuff of intrinsic tongue musculature to ensure biopsy extends well beyond the basement membrane.

(eg, MMP) cannot be detected without erosive lesion or "peeled" bed has no diagnostic value because the intraepithelial destruction (eg, PV) or subepithelial destruction (eg, MMP) cannot be detected without epithelium. Oral soft tissues affected by AIBD are often fragile and separation between the epithelium and underlying connective tissue ("peeling") is not uncommon. Precaution should be taken while performing a biopsy to avoid loss of epithelium. Local anesthetic injection can cause epithelium detachment before cutting the tissue and suction and vigorous blotting should be avoided during the biopsy. Oral biopsy should be performed by a skilled specialist who is experienced in the biopsy of AIBD lesions. Some practitioners favor a punch biopsy over scalpel biopsy, particularly on gingival tissue; however, it is the authors' opinion that it should be the decision of preforming specialists because many factors (eg, cutting force, depth control, accessibility, and the site of the biopsy) can affect the outcomes.[15]

Oral Brush Cytology

Although scalpel biopsy is considered to be the gold standard for definitive diagnosis of oral cancerous lesions, cytologic testing (eg, OralCDx, OralCyte, ClearPrep OC) has been marketed as a minimally invasive method to use as an adjunctive tool for screening and early detection of oral cancer.[16,17] OralCDx Brush Test has been available since 1999.[18] In performing this diagnostic test, a practitioner makes 10 to 20 rotations using a specialized brush to collect transepithelial cellular samples, which does not require a local anesthetic injection to the testing site. These samples fixed onto a glass slide are sent to a laboratory for staining, scanning, and analysis based on a computer-based imaging system to rank cells based on degree of abnormal morphology.[16] A cytopathologist interprets the results and reports as negative or benign, positive (defined as definitive cellular evidence of epithelial dysplasia or carcinoma), or atypical (defined as abnormal epithelial changes of uncertain diagnostic significance).[16] For all positive or atypical cases, a scalpel biopsy is recommended for a definitive diagnosis.[16]

A recent systematic review and meta-analysis found cytologic testing to be the most accurate adjunct for the evaluation of potentially malignant disorders in the oral cavity among those included in the review (autofluorescence, tissue reflectance, and vital staining).[17] Yet, the authors raised the concerns of the high rate of false-positive results and serious issues of risk of bias.

Although different cytopathology techniques have emerged in the past several years to improve sensitivity of the brush cytology, clinicians should note that scalpel biopsy by experts followed by a histopathology review is the single method leading to the definitive diagnosis of oral cancer to date.[16,19] Brush cytology is not recommended for lesions that are clinically suspicious for representing cancer.

SUMMARY

Biopsy of oral mucosal lesions is a procedure that is safely performed in most cases in the outpatient ambulatory setting using local anesthesia. Special considerations should be taken depending on the presumed diagnosis based on physical examination.

DISCLOSURE

Authors have nothing to disclose.

REFERENCES

1. Hurkudli DS, Sarvajnamurthy S, Suryanarayan S, et al. Novel uses of skin biopsy punches in dermatosurgery. Indian J Dermatol 2015;60:170.
2. H Alsarraf A, Kujan O, Farah CS. The utility of oral brush cytology in the early detection of oral cancer and oral potentially malignant disorders: a systematic review. J Oral Pathol Med 2018;47:104.
3. Navone R, Burlo P, Pich A, et al. The impact of liquid-based oral cytology on the diagnosis of oral squamous dysplasia and carcinoma. Cytopathology 2007;18:356.
4. Orosco RK, Tapia VJ, Califano JA, et al. Positive surgical margins in the 10 most common solid cancers. Sci Rep 2018;8:5686.
5. Sim YC, Hwang JH, Ahn KM. Overall and disease-specific survival outcomes following primary surgery for oral squamous cell carcinoma: analysis of consecutive 67- patients. J Korean Assoc Oral Maxillofac Surg 2019;45:83–90.
6. Shanti RM, O'Malley BW Jr. Surgical management of oral cancer. Dent Clin North Am 2018;62:77.
7. Shah J. Patters of cervical lymph node metastasis from squamous carcinomas of the upper aerodigestive tract. Am J Surg 1990;160:405–9.
8. Kane SV, Gupta M, Kakade AC, et al. Depth of invasion is the most significant histological predictor of subclinical cervical lymph node metastasis in early squamous cell carcinoma of the oral cavity. Eur J Surg Oncol 2006;32:795–803.
9. Mizrachi A, Migliacci JC, Montero PH, et al. Neck recurrence in clinically node-negative oral cancer: 27-year experience at a single institution. Oral Oncol 2018;78:94–101.
10. Chan LS, Ahmed AR, Anhalt GJ, et al. The first international consensus on mucous membrane

pemphigoid: definition, diagnostic criteria, pathogenic factors, medical treatment, and prognostic indicators. Arch Dermatol 2002;138(3):370–9.

11. Buonavoglia A, Leone P, Dammacco R, et al. Pemphigus and mucous membrane pemphigoid: an update from diagnosis to therapy. Autoimmun Rev 2019;18(4):349–58.

12. Rashid H, Lamberts A, Diercks GFH, et al. Oral lesions in autoimmune bullous diseases: an overview of clinical characteristics and diagnostic algorithm. Am J Clin Dermatol 2019;20(6):847–61.

13. The International Pemphigus & Pemphigoid Foundation's website. Available at: http://www.pemphigus.org/awareness/for-dental-professionals-students/biopsy/.

14. Kamaguchi M, Iwata H, Ujiie I, et al. Direct immunofluorescence using non-lesional buccal mucosa in mucous membrane pemphigoid. Front Med (Lausanne) 2018;5:20. The international pemphigus & pemphigoid foundation's website: Available at: http://www.pemphigus.org/awareness/for-dental-professionals-students/biopsy/.

15. Gilvetti C, Collyer J, Gulati A, et al. What is the optimal site and biopsy technique for the diagnosis of oral mucosal autoimmune blistering disease? J Oral Pathol Med 2019;48(3):239–43.

16. Patton LL1, Epstein JB, Kerr AR. Adjunctive techniques for oral cancer examination and lesion diagnosis: a systematic review of the literature. J Am Dent Assoc 2008;139(7):896–905.

17. Lingen MW, Tampi MP, Urquhart O, et al. Adjuncts for the evaluation of potentially malignant disorders in the oral cavity: diagnostic test accuracy systematic review and meta-analysis-a report of the American Dental Association. J Am Dent Assoc 2017;148(11):797–813.

18. Bhoopathi V, Kabani S, Mascarenhas AK. Low positive predictive value of the oral brush biopsy in detecting dysplastic oral lesions. Cancer 2009;115(5):1036–40.

19. Carreras-Torras C, Gay-Escoda C. Techniques for early diagnosis of oral squamous cell carcinoma: systematic review. Med Oral Patol Oral Cir Bucal 2015;20(3):e305–15.

Oral Granulomatous Disease

Faizan Alawi, DDS[a],*, Bridget E. Shields, MD[b], Temitope Omolehinwa, DMD[c],
Misha Rosenbach, MD[b]

KEYWORDS

- Foreign body reaction • Crohn disease • Sarcoidosis • Infectious disease
- Orofacial granulomatosis • Periorificial dermatitis • Granulomatosis with polyangiitis

KEY POINTS

- Granulomatous diseases are a heterogeneous group of chronic inflammatory disorders whose pathogenesis is triggered by an array of infectious and noninfectious agents.
- Granulomatous diseases may be localized or a manifestation of systemic, disseminated disease, and often present in the oral soft tissues with nonspecific signs and symptoms.
- Identifying the underlying cause of the inflammation may be challenging, and often requires correlation of clinical, microscopic, and laboratory findings.

INTRODUCTION

Granulomatous inflammation is a type IV, delayed-type hypersensitivity reaction to an array of infectious and noninfectious agents, and may be localized or present as systemic, disseminated disease.[1] Granulomas are composed primarily of macrophages (epithelioid histiocytes) accompanied by multinucleated giant cells and predominantly CD4+ T lymphocytes (**Fig. 1**).[2] The primary functions of the histiocytes are to phagocytose foreign material or microorganisms; antigen presentation; and secretion of chemokines, cytokines, and other chemotactic mediators to further propagate the inflammatory reaction.

Macrophage polarization is important in the pathogenesis of granulomatous disease.[2] M1 macrophages are classically activated by cytokines such as interleukin-2, interferon-γ, and tumor necrosis factor (TNF)-α, and primarily participate in microbial killing; M1 macrophages accumulate early in disease.[2] In contrast, M2 macrophages (alternatively activated macrophages) often appear late or in resolving disease states,

express antiinflammatory cytokines, and primarily contribute to immunoregulation and tissue modeling, including fibrosis.[2]

The causes of oral granulomatous disease are similar to those that induce cutaneous disease.[2] Infectious causes mostly include mycobacterial and fungal organisms. Noninfectious sources of granulomatous inflammation include foreign materials, environmental antigens, circulating metabolites, and malignancy.[3] In the absence of overt foreign material or a recognizable infectious agent, identifying the underlying cause of the inflammation can be challenging.[1] This article highlights various conditions associated with granulomatous inflammation within the oral and perioral soft tissues.

FOREIGN BODY REACTION

Foreign material, including an array of dental materials and cosmetic fillers, is the most common source of oral granulomatous disorder.[1,3,4] Patients typically present with nonspecific features, including persistent or intermittent lip, buccal

[a] Department of Basic and Translational Sciences, University of Pennsylvania School of Dental Medicine, 240 South 40th Street, Philadelphia, PA 19104, USA; [b] Department of Dermatology, Hospital of the University of Pennsylvania, 3400 Civic Center Blvd, Philadelphia, PA 19104, USA; [c] Department of Oral Medicine, University of Pennsylvania School of Dental Medicine, 240 South 40th Street, Philadelphia, PA 19104, USA
* Corresponding author.
E-mail address: falawi@upenn.edu

Dermatol Clin 38 (2020) 429–439
https://doi.org/10.1016/j.det.2020.05.004

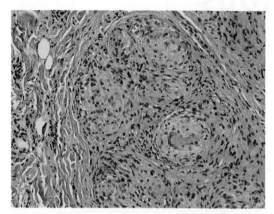

Fig. 1. Noncaseous granulomas (hematoxylin-eosin, original magnification ×200).

mucosa, or gingival swelling, which could be localized to the area of foreign body impaction or more diffuse.[1] Rarely, patients present with solitary or diffuse ulcerations. Biopsy is required for definitive diagnosis, especially because the inflammatory response may occur many months to years from the time of exposure to the foreign body, and patients may not recall exposure to the substance.[1]

On microscopic identification of granulomas within biopsy tissue, the presence of foreign material should be investigated under visible light and through the use of polarized light to identify a potentially birefringent substance (**Fig. 2**).[1] However, the inability to identify foreign material does not preclude this as a potential cause of the inflammatory pattern. Similarly, the presence of foreign material does not preempt a diagnosis of systemic causality. Foreign bodies are occasionally identified in cutaneous biopsies obtained from patients with sarcoidosis, a systemic granulomatous

disease.[5] Removal of the foreign material with or without use of a topical or intralesional steroid should resolve the signs and symptoms.[1]

PERIORAL/PERIORIFICIAL DERMATITIS

Perioral dermatitis is a localized inflammatory process consisting of papules and pustules symmetrically distributed around the mouth.[6] A characteristic zone of clearing beyond the vermilion border is often present.[6] Crops of grouped, follicular, pink-red papules, papulovesicles, and pustules may recur over weeks to months and be accompanied by fine scaling.[7] When periorbital or perinasal locations are involved, the term periorificial dermatitis is favored. About 90% of cases occur in women (ages 16–45 years) and children.[6,8] Cases of perioral dermatitis occurring in men are estimated to increase because of shifting cosmetic practices.[7] Granulomatous periorificial dermatitis (GPD) is a distinct granulomatous variant seen most frequently in prepubertal children or patients with darker skin phenotypes. Clinically, granulomatous lesions may show yellow coloration on diascopy. Patients are typically asymptomatic but may report irritation or a burning sensation. Lesions are rarely pruritic.

Fluorinated or nonfluorinated topical corticosteroid use preceding the eruption is frequently identified. Use may be in the form of inhaled corticosteroids or prescription topicals.[8] Fluorinated toothpaste; overuse of heavy cosmetic creams; and the use of petrolatum, paraffin, or isopropyl myristate (a vehicle in many topicals) have also been implicated.[7] Additional causes of perioral dermatitis are outlined in **Table 1**. Histopathology of early lesions can show epidermal acanthosis, parakeratosis, and edema with

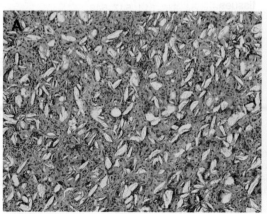
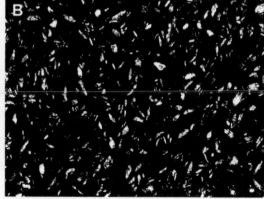

Fig. 2. (A) Diffuse granulomatous inflammation with optically clear foreign material dispersed throughout (hematoxylin-eosin, original magnification ×100). (B) The material birefringed under polarized light (original magnification×100).

Table 1
Causes of perioral dermatitis

Drugs	• Topical steroids • Inhaled prescription steroid sprays (fluorinated and nonfluorinated)
Cosmetics	• Fluorinated toothpaste • Skin care ointments and creams • Mercury-containing dental fillings • Mint-flavored tooth-cleaning powder
Physical factors	• Ultraviolet light • Heat • Wind
Microbiologic factors	• Fusiform spirilla bacteria • *Candida* species • *Demodex folliculorum*
Miscellaneous factors	• Hormonal factors (oral contraceptives) • Gastrointestinal disturbances (malabsorption) • Emotional stress • Musical instruments • Latex gloves • Lipstick • Response to permethrin treatment

From Lipozenčić J, Hadžavdić SL. Perioral dermatitis. Clin Dermatol. 2014;32(1):125-130.; with permission.

underlying perivascular and perifollicular lympho-histiocytic infiltration.[8] Late papular lesions and GPD variant may reveal discrete, noncaseating, epithelioid granulomas distributed perifollicularly and with surrounding lymphocytic inflammation. Caseating granulomas may be seen in GPD.[7] However, many patients with periorificial derma-titis are treated with topical corticosteroids, which initially improve the eruption but result in disease recurrence, often worse than the primary derma-titis. Discontinuation of any triggering medication is the first step in management. Additional thera-pies are outlined in **Table 2**.

INFECTIOUS DISEASE

Several infectious organisms trigger a granuloma-tous inflammatory reaction.[1] Pathologists con-fronted with granulomatous inflammation within biopsy tissue should obtain Gomori methenamine silver nitrate and periodic acid–Schiff histologic stains to identify potential fungal organisms, and a Ziehl-Neelsen stain to highlight acid-fast organisms, namely mycobacterial species.[1] How-ever, negative findings with any of these analyses do not preclude an infectious cause and additional laboratory testing, including molecular studies such as polymerase chain reaction (PCR) and/or cultures, may be warranted. Prototypical exam-ples of infection-related, orofacial granulomatous disease are described later.

TUBERCULOSIS

Orofacial tuberculosis (TB) is a rare form of extrap-ulmonary TB accounting for only 0.05% to 5% of all cases of TB.[9] Classically caused by *Mycobac-terium tuberculosis* (MBT) complex, orofacial TB represents the prototypical infection-induced granulomatous disease.[1] Orofacial TB can be pri-mary (with the oral mucosa as the initial site of infection) or secondary (internal organ TB with subsequent autoinoculation orally).[10] Secondary involvement is seen more frequently, especially in adults.[9,11] Most reported cases of oral TB are the result of direct mucosal contact with infected sputum where invasion of the submucosal tissue is made possible by preceding mucosal trauma.[12,13]

Oral lesions may be present before systemic symptoms, making awareness of orofacial TB especially important for physicians and dentists alike.[14] Orofacial TB can involve the entire oral cavity, including the lips, oral mucosa, tongue, pal-ate, sinuses, maxillary and mandibular bones, and temporomandibular joints.[14] The tongue is the location most commonly affected.[11] Clinical pre-sentation can be highly variable and patients may show persistent, painful, ulceration, gingivitis (nodular or papillary proliferations and hyperemia of the gingival tissue), osteomyelitis, sialadenitis, lymphadenitis, or periapical granulomatous dis-ease. Painful cervical lymphadenopathy may accompany any form of the disease.[10] The devel-opment of sentinel tubercles (small nodules sur-rounding tuberculous ulcerations) may be a clue to diagnosis.[14] Intraosseous TB of the maxillary and mandibular bones, as well as tuberculous granulation tissue, have been reported following dental extraction where sockets serve as a route of organism entry.[9,12,14]

Classification criteria for orofacial TB have been proposed based on the anatomic location involved; these criteria have not yet been widely accepted.[13] Lupus vulgaris may present with brown to yellow granulomatous lesions surround-ing facial orifices.[15] A high index of suspicion is key to making the diagnosis of orofacial TB. Treatment-nonresponsive, persistent, or fistulous lesions should be biopsied. Early lesions and

Table 2
Therapeutic agents for periorificial dermatitis

Topical Agents	Level of Evidence[a]	Systemic Agents	Level of Evidence[a]
Metronidazole	A	Tetracycline	A
Erythromycin	A	Erythromycin	D
Pimecrolimus	A	Doxycycline	D
Sulfacetamide or sulfur	B	Minocycline	D
Azelaic acid	B	Cefcapene pivoxil hydrochloride hydrate	D
Clindamycin	C	Isotretinoin	D
Tacrolimus	D	Other	—
Adapalene	D	Zero therapy	A
—	—	PDL	C

[a] A, high-quality randomized controlled trial (RCT) or prospective study; B, lesser-quality RCT or prospective study; C, case-control study or retrospective study; D, case series or case reports.
From Lee GL, Zirwas MJ. Granulomatous Rosacea and Periorificial Dermatitis: Controversies and Review of Management and Treatment. Dermatol Clin. 2015;33(3):447-455.; with permission.

immunocompromised patients may lack the classic, deep dermal, caseating granulomatous inflammation expected of MBT.[11] Although microscopic confirmation of acid-fast microorganisms is confirmatory of orofacial TB, many prior studies suggest that only a small percentage of specimens stain positively, requiring tissue culture.[1,11] PCR, tuberculin skin testing, and interferon-γ release assays may all support the diagnosis.

Although MBT serves as the prototypical example of orofacial granulomatous disease, similar diseases may be caused by other mycobacterial organisms, including *Mycobacterium bovis*, *Mycobacterium leprae*, *Mycobacterium avium* complex, and *Mycobacterium marinum*.[1] Treatment of orofacial TB is often challenging, especially as drug-resistant TB emerges, and should be undertaken with the assistance of infectious disease physicians.

HISTOPLASMOSIS

Histoplasmosis is an infection caused by the saprophytic and dimorphic fungus, *Histoplasma capsulatum*.[16] Histoplasmosis occurs in 3 forms: acute, chronic, and disseminated.[17] Rarely, direct inoculation occurs. Multiorgan dissemination often arises in immunocompromised hosts.[18] Mucosal sites are preferentially involved (and may serve as the first and only sign of disease) when dissemination occurs.[17] Between 20% and 50% of patients reportedly show oral lesions in the setting of systemic disease.[19] Rarely, localized lesions of the oral mucosa without dissemination and in immunocompetent patients have been reported.[16]

Oral ulcerations are the most common lesions encountered and are typically deep seated and painful.[17] Oral cavity histoplasmosis may also show nodular, plaquelike, or vegetative morphology, and can localize to the tongue, palate, and buccal mucosa.

Histopathologic findings may include noncaseating granulomatous inflammation with macrophages containing 2-μm to 4-μm, grouped, narrow-based budding yeasts with a clear zone corresponding with the cell wall.[18] Demonstration of *H capsulatum* on histopathology or culture are the gold standards for definitive diagnosis. Antigenuria and/or antigenemia and positive serologies may support the diagnosis.[20]

Other fungal infections that result in granulomatous inflammation of the oral mucosa include *Paracoccidioides brasiliensis*, *Cryptococcus neoformans*, *Coccidioides immitis*, and *Blastomyces dermatitidis*, which can all induce similar disease.[1] Treatment of histoplasmosis depends on the degree of systemic involvement and host immune status, and infectious disease consultation is advised. Severe, disseminated disease is typically treated with intravenous, lipid formulation of amphotericin B (3.0–5.0 mg/kg/d) followed by itraconazole.[20] Patients with mild disease and normal immunity may be treated with itraconazole alone (200–600 mg/d). Voriconazole and posaconazole have also be used successfully.[20]

SYPHILIS

Syphilis is a sexually or vertically transmitted chronic infection caused by the anaerobic spirochete *Treponema pallidum*.[21] Syphilis progresses through primary and secondary stages followed by late or unknown-duration syphilis, as well as a latent period of variable length.[21] Oral lesions may be present in any syphilitic stage.[22] In 2018, a rate of 10.8 cases of syphilis per 100,000 people was reported in the United States, an increase from previous years.[23] Worldwide, more than 5 million new cases of syphilis are diagnosed each year.[24]

Primary syphilis presents between 3 and 90 days following inoculation and is characterized by an asymptomatic papule that ulcerates to form a chancre at the site of infection.[21,24] Although the primary chancre heals over 3 to 6 weeks without treatment, the organism is subsequently disseminated via lymphatic or hematogenous spread, resulting in secondary syphilis.[24] The secondary stage of disease is characterized by heterogeneous clinical manifestations involving the skin and mucosae, involved in 90% to 97% of cases.[21] Accompanying fever, malaise, pharyngitis, and generalized lymphadenopathy may be present.[21,24] Mucosal syphilis may be present in one-third to one-half of patients with secondary syphilis, and may include so-called mucous patches (ovoid, ulcerative or erythematous, thin, white plaques with surrounding erythema or serpiginous, snail-tracking ulceration) or leukoplakialike plaques (verrucous lesions).[21,22,25] Split papules (fausse syphilitic perlèche or false angular cheilitis) may present at the commissures.[25] Lesion distribution can include the hard palate, lips, buccal mucosa, and tongue.[22] Glossodynia and tonsillitis as the sole manifestations of secondary syphilis have been described.[25,26] Late-duration syphilis may involve the oral mucosa and present as gummatous lesions or as atrophic luetic glossitis.[27]

Because *T pallidum* cannot be cultured, treponemal and nontreponemal serologies are often used.[28] Histopathologic features of syphilis depend on the lesion biopsied and the stage of disease. Epithelial acanthosis with basovacuolar change may exist.[28] Inflammation within the lamina propria with perivascular lymphocytes, histiocytes, and plasma cells is often present. Endothelial cell swelling and proliferation are characteristic.[28] Granulomatous inflammation is a hallmark of late-duration syphilis and may show associated caseative necrosis.[28] Identification of spirochetes in formalin-fixed tissue is best achieved with immunohistochemical stains using antibodies to treponemal antigens.[28] Benzathine penicillin G is the treatment of choice for all stages of syphilis. Disease stage, pregnancy status, allergies, and organ involvement determine duration and route of administration.[28]

CROHN DISEASE

Crohn disease (CD) is a chronic, relapsing, inflammatory bowel disorder that can affect any portion of the digestive tract, from the mouth to the anus, and usually with discontinuous skip lesions.[29] CD is thought to arise from an alteration in the intestinal microbiome or disruption of the mucosal epithelium, which normally equilibrate the response to these organisms.[30] CD has an annual incidence rate of 3 to 20 per 100,000 with a bimodal age of onset, and a prevalence of approximately 200 per 100,000.[31] Most patients initially present with disease between the second and fourth decades of life. A smaller subset of patients begins developing disease around the age of 50 years. Overall, the disease is more prevalent in individuals of Ashkenazi Jewish origin, and in North America and Western Europe, compared with other populations, but the incidence seems to be increasing in Asia.[31] There is no distinct sex predilection. Current classification of CD is based on the age of initial diagnosis, anatomic location of the intestinal disease, and clinical behavior of the disease.[31]

Genetic, immunologic, and environmental factors contribute to CD risk and pathogenesis.[31] A family history of CD is identified in up to 15% of patients with CD and concordance rates in monozygotic twins ranges from 20% to 50%.[29] Several genes have been linked to CD but the strongest associations are with nucleotide-binding oligomerization domain–containing protein 2 (*NOD2*), autophagy-related 16-like 1 (*ATG16L1*), and interleukin-23 receptor (*IL23R*).[30] These factors are implicated in regulation of autophagy, innate immunity, and bacterial sensing.[30] Patients with CD have a reduced diversity in their gut microbiome compared with healthy individuals.[30] The mechanisms remain poorly understood, but this dysbiosis may also increase the risk for CD. Other environmental risk factors include smoking, history of low-fiber and high-fatty-acid diets, sustained use of nonsteroidal antiinflammatory medications, contraceptive usage, and early childhood antibiotic treatment, such as with doxycycline.[31]

It is estimated that up to one-third of all patients with CD experience at least 1 extraintestinal manifestation, including oral lesions, at some point during the course of their disease.[32] In up to 60% of patients with CD, oral manifestations may precede gastrointestinal signs and symptoms.[33] In pediatric patients, oral manifestations have been reported in up to 80% of reported cohorts.[34] Moreover, the younger the onset, the more likely it is to be a male patient.[35] The signs and symptoms of CD are highly variable and can be divided into specific and nonspecific manifestations.[32,34,36] The most common sites of involvement are the lips, gingiva, and mucobuccal folds. Intermittent painless swelling of 1 or both lips; generalized gingival erythema and edema (**Fig. 3**); linear ulcerations, often with hyperplastic folds located in the vestibular sulci; mucosal cobblestoning; and tissue tags are some of the most common specific oral manifestations.[33,36] Aphthous stomatitis and xerostomia are examples of nonspecific manifestations.[32,33] A systematic review of the literature revealed lip swelling as the presenting sign in most pediatric patients.[37]

Diagnosis of CD is made primarily through clinical, endoscopic, pathologic, and radiographic evaluation, accompanied by laboratory testing, including serology and other nonspecific analyses.[29] On histology, noncaseating granulomas may be seen in up to 50% of tissue biopsies, and may be confirmatory of disease when identified in patients with classic signs and symptoms.

A diffuse and dense inflammatory infiltrate composed of lymphocytes, plasma cells, mast cells, and occasional eosinophils is also frequently seen. The inflammation often extends deep into the submucosal tissue.

Treatment varies depending on the severity, location, and clinical subtype of disease and may require medical and surgical intervention.[29] Topical therapy with corticosteroids can be useful in mild cases or as an adjunctive measure. For patients with oral and systemic manifestations, medical management may be with immunosuppressants such as prednisone, methotrexate, and/or biologic drugs, many of which target TNF-α.[31] Thiopurines such as 6-mercaptopurine or azathioprine are often used for long-term control. Oral prednisone as a monotherapy may be beneficial in patients who manifest with disease limited to the oral cavity. A patient with severe refractory oral CD was successfully treated with ustekinumab.[38] Ustekinumab is a monoclonal antibody to the p-40 subunit of interleukin-12 and interleukin-

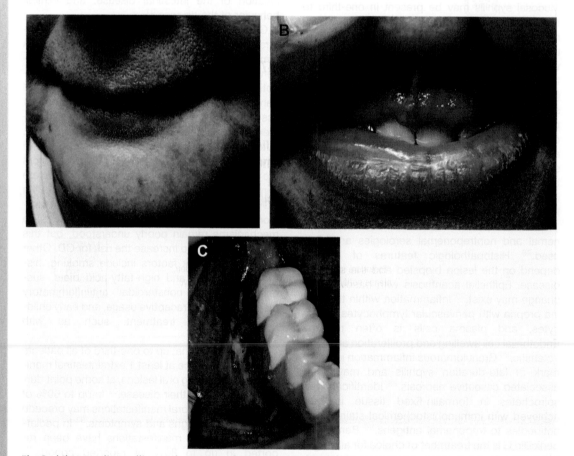

Fig. 3. (*A*) Upper lip swelling in the setting of quiescent CD. (*B*) Extensive gingival hypertrophy as a manifestation of previously undiagnosed, untreated Crohn disease. (*C*) Linear ulceration in the mandibular lingual vestibule (*arrows*).

23 and was recently approved for use in patients with moderate to severe CD. Intralesional corticosteroid injections may aid in resolution of persistent fixed or resistant lesions.

SARCOIDOSIS

Sarcoidosis is a multisystem inflammatory disease of unknown cause characterized by the development of noncaseating granulomas in multiple organ systems.[39] The skin is involved in 25% to 35% of cases, although the prevalence of mucosal disease is less well characterized. Sarcoidosis is a protean disease, and mucocutaneous involvement may present with multiple, varied clinical morphologies.

Head and neck involvement occurs in 10% to 15% of cases,[40] although oral sarcoidosis itself is rare, with fewer than 100 well-documented cases in the English literature.[41] However, because the lesions are often nonspecific in appearance, oral sarcoidosis may be underreported. Oral involvement may occur concurrent with systemic disease or as the initial manifestation in some cases, potentially preceding systemic involvement by years. In approximately one-quarter of reported cases of oral involvement, sarcoidosis affected the bone of the jaws and led to loose teeth, pain, mandibular swelling, and non-healing socket.[42] Direct involvement of the soft tissues can occur as well, most commonly with lesions on the buccal mucosa. Signs and symptoms can include swelling, papules, nodules, erosions/ulcers, gingival hyperplasia, recession, or gingivitis (**Fig. 4**). Sarcoidosis may affect the lips, gingiva, floor of the mouth, hard and/or soft palate, tongue, or vestibule, and can also involve the adenoids, uvula, or posterior oropharynx. Classically, oral sarcoidal lesions are asymptomatic, well-circumscribed, brown-red or violaceous papules, plaques, or nodules.

Although oral mucosal sarcoidosis is rare, salivary gland involvement is common, and may present with xerostomia. Salivary gland biopsy from clinically normal tissue may show sarcoidal granulomas up to 60% of the time.[41] Symptomatic disease may present with parotid swelling (including Heerfordt syndrome, characterized by parotid swelling, uveitis, and facial nerve palsy), submandibular lymphadenopathy, and/or xerostomia. Salivary gland biopsy may be required to distinguish sarcoidosis from Sjögren syndrome.

Patients with suspected sarcoidosis should undergo a thorough, multidisciplinary evaluation for systemic disease. This evaluation typically includes pulmonary radiography; basic laboratory tests, including evaluation for hypercalcemia and electrocardiogram (ECG); a thorough review of systems with targeted additional work-up, including cardiac evaluation if there are palpitations or ECG abnormalities; plus an ophthalmologic evaluation. Serum angiotensin-converting enzyme level may be increased in sarcoidosis but is neither sensitive nor specific, although levels more than 2 to 3 times the upper limit may be suggestive. A biopsy of affected tissue is generally

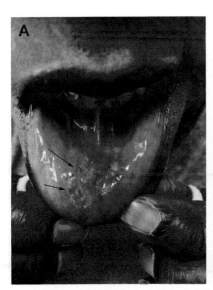
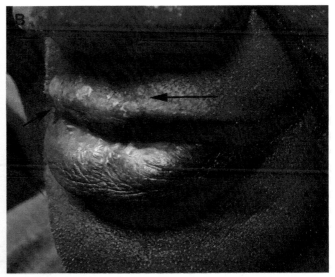

Fig. 4. (A) Sclerotic, dyspigmented, slightly erythematous patch (*arrows*) was the sole oral mucosal involvement of this patient's multiorgan sarcoidosis (skin, lungs). (B) Different patient with flesh-colored to slightly erythematous flat papules (*arrows*) across the mucocutaneous border and vermilion lip, extending up to the philtrum.

suggested, because supportive histopathology showing noncaseating granulomas (**Fig. 5**) and excluding infection and other mimickers is important in making the diagnosis.

The differential diagnosis includes entities discussed throughout this article, and physicians should take care to exclude CD, granulomatosis with polyangiitis, foreign body granulomas, and Melkersson-Rosenthal syndrome.

Treatment is generally directed at the most severely affected organ. Oral sarcoidosis may not require treatment. Mild cases may be treated with topical or intralesional corticosteroids, or more widespread disease may require antiinflammatory treatment (hydroxychloroquine, tetracycline-class antibiotics), or immunosuppressive treatment in severe cases (systemic corticosteroids, methotrexate, TNF inhibitors, or other agents).[43]

OROFACIAL GRANULOMATOSIS

Orofacial granulomatosis (OFG) is a diagnosis of exclusion, because all other systemic granulomatous conditions have to be ruled out radiographically, clinically, by endoscopy, and via serology to come to a diagnosis.[44] When OFG is diagnosed in pediatric patients, long-term monitoring is important, because OFG can be an early sign of CD. Bowel involvement has been reported in up to one-third of patients with OFG.[45] Overall, there is no gender or ethnic predilection, with median age of onset around the second to third decade of life.[46] Clinical variants of OFG include:

1. Melkersson-Rosenthal syndrome: patients with this condition present with idiopathic OFG, fissured tongue, and Bell palsy.
2. Cheilitis granulomatosa of Miescher: persistent lip swelling is the only manifestation noted in patients with cheilitis granulomatosa.

The cause of OFG remains largely unknown, which is possibly a result of disease rarity. However, a weak genetic association has been suspected, because human leukocyte antigen (HLA)-B16 and HLA-CW$_3$ have been identified in some patients with Melkersson-Rosenthal syndrome.[47] Food products, dental hygiene products and dental materials, immunomodulation, and microbial infections have also been implicated as possible causes; cinnamon, chocolate, cocoa, and benzoate are the most commonly associated.[44]

The most prevalent clinical feature associated with OFG is labial swelling (**Fig. 6**), and this is present in more than 90% of patients with disease. Note that this swelling/edematous presentation of the lips when palpated does not trigger a painful response or discomfort. The swelling is also

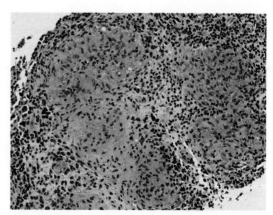

Fig. 5. Granulomatous inflammation in a patient with intraosseous mandibular sarcoidosis (hematoxylin-eosin, original magnification ×200).

nonpitting and does not affect patients' speech. OFG may present as intermittent or persistent soft labial swelling, especially during the initial phase of presentation, or doughy, firm, or indurated labial swelling as the disease progresses. There may be gingival, floor-of-the mouth, and/or buccal mucosa swelling and/or erythema in the presence of the labial swelling, and, rarely, nonspecific extraoral or intraoral ulcers.[46] Facial palsy and fissured tongue (lingua plicata) in the

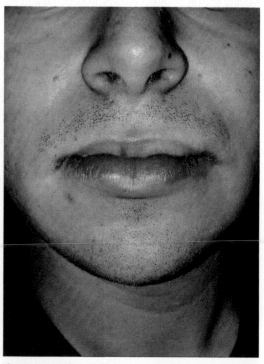

Fig. 6. Lower lip swelling as a manifestation of orofacial granulomatosis. This patient also presented with angular cheilitis.

presence of labial swelling is often noted in Melkersson-Rosenthal syndrome. The facial palsy is thought to be as a result of granulomatous infiltration of the nerve sheath or compression of the nerves from the swelling. OFG may also involve other nonoral sites, including the cheek, forehead, and periorbital region.[48]

A biopsy is warranted for diagnosis and typically reveals noncaseating granulomas.[46] However, the diagnosis is one of exclusion, after ruling out other causes of systemic granulomatosis, and no cause can be identified. Patch testing may be needed to rule out an allergic reaction.

Treatment of OFG is usually esthetic, and includes the injection of intralesional steroids. Topical steroids can be applied to intraoral lesions, including areas with erythema and ulceration. Systemic corticosteroids have also been used, although there are risks involved in long-term use of steroids. Surgical debulking may be necessary if the swelling does not resolve with local therapy, as previously mentioned. Some patients are also prescribed antifungal or antibacterial agents if an infectious cause is suspected. In addition, biologic agents such as adalimumab, injected subcutaneously, and dapsone (or a combination of dapsone and steroids) have been used.

GRANULOMATOSIS WITH POLYANGIITIS

Rare lymphomas, including Hodgkin disease and some T-cell lymphomas, may also present with granulomatous inflammation in conjunction with the malignant lymphoid proliferation; the mechanisms remain poorly understood.[49,50] However, despite the presence of granulomatous inflammation, these malignancies are not considered granulomatous diseases. Similarly, granulomatous inflammation may also be observed in systemic diseases, including small vessel vasculitides.[51] One disease merits inclusion in this article because it may be included in the differential diagnosis of many of the conditions described earlier.

Granulomatosis with polyangiitis (GPA), previously known as Wegener granulomatosis, is a destructive and progressive, multiorgan autoimmune disease.[51] GPA is characterized by inflammation of small blood vessel walls (vasculitis) and the presence of circulating antineutrophil cytoplasmic antibodies (ANCAs) to either proteinase 3 (PR3), also called myeloblastin, or myeloperoxidase (MPO). GPA is more commonly associated with PR3-ANCA than MPO-ANCA.[51] Patients typically present with disease after the age of 50 years, with a peak incidence rate between the ages of 60 and 70 years. Overall, GPA affects 6 to 12 per million population.[52]

ANCAs serve not only as a disease biomarker but also in pathogenesis.[51] PR3 and MPO are contained in neutrophils within primary cytoplasmic granules. Following infection or inflammation, proinflammatory cytokines such as interleukin-1 and TNF-α, complement C5a, and lipopolysaccharide prime neutrophils, thereby inducing movement of MPO and PR3 to the cell surface.[53] ANCAs then bind to their autoantigens, leading to vigorous neutrophil activation. The neutrophils then bind to vascular endothelium to induce the vasculitis.

The mechanisms by which GPA-associated ANCAs develop remains poorly understood. Genetic risk factors have been identified, most notably single nucleotide polymorphisms in proteinase 3 (PRTN3), SERPINA1 encoding α1-antitrypsin, which is the serine protease inhibitor of PR3, and HLA-DP.[53] Epidemiologic studies also suggest infection with Staphylococcus aureus or exposure to chemicals, including silica and hydrocarbons, may trigger disease in a subset of patients.[51]

GPA is a systemic, multiorgan disease often characterized by involvement with the upper and lower respiratory tracts and kidney.[51] Upper respiratory tract disease, which is the single most commonly encountered manifestation, may present as chronic, refractory sinusitis, rhinitis, epistaxis, or otitis media. Patients often complain of constitutional signs and symptoms, including fever, malaise, fatigue, and unexplained weight loss, often for months before more overt manifestations become apparent. Nonspecific cutaneous lesions may be observed in up to 50% of patients.[36] Oral manifestations may be more commonly encountered than skin lesions, and up to 6% of patients may manifest with oral lesions as their presenting complaint.[54] Oral manifestations are among the diagnostic criteria for GPA issued by American College of Rheumatology.[54]

Hyperplastic gingivitis is described as specific for GPA (**Fig. 7**), but it can occur in other entities (eg, leukemia).[55] Most commonly seen in the maxillary anterior gingiva, the hyperplastic tissue associated with GPA is painless, friable, edematous, and red-purple in coloration (similar color to strawberries). As a result, this feature is frequently described as strawberry gingivitis. Other oral pathology is nonspecific and may include painful ulceration, palatal necrosis, alveolar bone loss, tooth mobility, gingival recession, oroantral fistulae, and labial mucosal nodules.

Diagnosis of GPA is challenging and is often made through clinical, pathologic, and radiographic evaluation, accompanied by laboratory testing, including blood, serology, and urinalysis.[52] On histology, noncaseating granulomatous inflammation may be identified, accompanied by a diffuse and

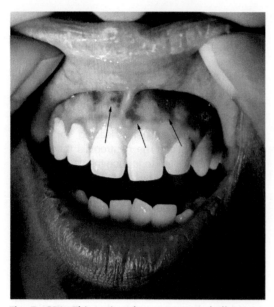

Fig. 7. GPA. This patient has numerous shallow erosions and maxillary gingival infiltration (*arrows*) during a flare of known GPA. She had a concurrent erosion on her posterior palate and small cutaneous ulceration on the right lower chin (not seen).

dense mixed inflammatory infiltrate composed of neutrophils, lymphocytes, plasma cells, and occasional eosinophils. More commonly, biopsy tissues reveal dense acute and chronic inflammation and extravasated hemorrhage but without granulomas. Leukocytoclastic vasculitis is observed in some tissue biopsies.

Immunosuppressive therapy using a combination of a glucocorticoid with cyclophosphamide or rituximab is often the initial approach to therapy.[51] Because of side effects and toxicity associated with prolonged use of cyclophosphamide, rituximab is preferable for some patients. Rituximab is also used in patients with relapsed disease.

SUMMARY

Identifying potential foreign material or possible infectious causes is usually the first approach when confronted with granulomatous inflammation. If absent, investigations that include clinical laboratory assessment of various markers that indicate infectious and systemic inflammatory disease, and other corollary tests, including serology, are often required. Appropriately diagnosing the cause of granulomatous inflammation often requires a multimodal and interdisciplinary approach.

DISCLOSURE

The authors have nothing to disclose.

REFERENCES

1. Alawi F. An update on granulomatous diseases of the oral tissues. Dent Clin North Am 2013;57(4):657–71.
2. Asai J. What is new in the histogenesis of granulomatous skin diseases? J Dermatol 2017;44(3):297–303.
3. Müller S. Non-infectious granulomatous lesions of the orofacial region. Head Neck Pathol 2019;13: 449–56.
4. Alcântara CEP, Noronha MS, Cunha JF, et al. Granulomatous reaction to hyaluronic acid filler material in oral and perioral region: A case report and review of literature. J Cosmet Dermatol 2018;17(4):578–83.
5. Marcoval J, Mañá J, Moreno A, et al. Foreign bodies in granulomatous cutaneous lesions of patients with systemic sarcoidosis. Arch Dermatol 2001;137(4): 427–30.
6. Lee GL, Zirwas MJ. Granulomatous Rosacea and Periorificial Dermatitis: Controversies and Review of Management and Treatment. Dermatol Clin 2015;33(3):447–55.
7. Lipozenčić J, Hadžavdić SL. Perioral dermatitis. Clin Dermatol 2014;32(1):125–30.
8. Lipozencic J, Ljubojevic S. Perioral dermatitis. Clin Dermatol 2011;29(2):157–61.
9. Mignogna MD, Muzio LL, Favia G, et al. Oral tuberculosis: a clinical evaluation of 42 cases. Oral Dis 2000;6(1):25–30.
10. Turkmen M, Turk BG, Kandıloglu G, et al. Tuberculosis cutis orificialis in an immunocompetent patient. Cutis 2015;95(2):E4–6.
11. Jain P, Jain I. Oral Manifestations of Tuberculosis: Step towards Early Diagnosis. J Clin Diagn Res 2014;8(12):ZE18–21.
12. Rinaggio J. Tuberculosis. Dent Clin North Am 2003; 47(3):449–65, v.
13. Andrade NN, Mhatre TS. Orofacial tuberculosis–a 16-year experience with 46 cases. J Oral Maxillofac Surg 2012;70(1):e12–22.
14. Bansal R, Jain A, Mittal S. Orofacial tuberculosis: Clinical manifestations, diagnosis and management. J Fam Med Prim Care 2015;4(3):335–41.
15. Pai VV, Naveen KN, Athanikar SB, et al. A clinico-histopathological study of lupus vulgaris: A 3 year experience at a tertiary care centre. Indian Dermatol Online J 2014;5(4):461–5.
16. O'Connell Ferster AP, Jaworek A, Hu A. Histoplasmosis of the head and neck in the immunocompetent patient: Report of 2 cases. Ear Nose Throat J 2018;97(9):E28–31.
17. Folk GA, Nelson BL. Oral Histoplasmosis. Head Neck Pathol 2017;11(4):513–6.
18. Guarner J, Brandt ME. Histopathologic diagnosis of fungal infections in the 21st century. Clin Microbiol Rev 2011;24(2):247–80.
19. Akin L, Herford AS, Cicciù M. Oral presentation of disseminated histoplasmosis: a case report and

literature review. J Oral Maxillofac Surg 2011;69(2): 535–41.

20. Wheat LJ, Freifeld AG, Kleiman MB, et al. Clinical practice guidelines for the management of patients with histoplasmosis: 2007 update by the Infectious Diseases Society of America. Clin Infect Dis 2007; 45(7):807–25.

21. Forrestel AK, Kovarik CL, Katz KA. Sexually acquired syphilis: Historical aspects, microbiology, epidemiology, and clinical manifestations. J Am Acad Dermatol 2020;82(1):1–14.

22. de Paulo LF, Servato JP, Oliveira MT, et al. Oral Manifestations of Secondary Syphilis. Int J Infect Dis 2015;35:40–2.

23. CDC.gov- Syphilis. 2018. Available at: https://www.cdc. gov/std/syphilis/stats.htm. Accessed January 8, 2020.

24. Hook EW. Syphilis. Lancet 2017;389(10078):1550–7.

25. Eyer-Silva WA, Freire MAL, Horta-Araujo CA, et al. Secondary Syphilis Presenting as Glossodynia. Case Rep Med 2017;2017:1980798.

26. Hamlyn E, Marriott D, Gallagher RM. Secondary syphilis presenting as tonsillitis in three patients. J Laryngol Otol 2006;120(7):602–4.

27. Leão JC, Gueiros LA, Porter SR. Oral manifestations of syphilis. Clinics (Sao Paulo) 2006;61(2):161–6.

28. Forrestel AK, Kovarik CL, Katz KA. Sexually acquired syphilis: Laboratory diagnosis, management, and prevention. J Am Acad Dermatol 2020;82(1): 17–28.

29. Feuerstein JD, Cheifetz AS. Crohn disease: epidemiology, diagnosis, and management. Mayo Clin Proc 2017;92(7):1088–103.

30. Stange EF, Schroeder BO. Microbiota and mucosal defense in IBD: an update. Expert Rev Gastroenterol Hepatol 2019;13(10):963–76.

31. Gajendran M, Loganathan P, Catinella AP, et al. A comprehensive review and update on Crohn's disease. Dis Mon 2018;64(2):20–57.

32. de Vries SAG, Tan CXW, Bouma G, et al. Salivary function and oral health problems in Crohn's disease patients. Inflamm Bowel Dis 2018;24(6):1361–7.

33. Lankarani KB, Sivandzadeh GR, Hassanpour S. Oral manifestation in inflammatory bowel disease: a review. World J Gastroenterol 2013;19(46):8571–9.

34. Eckel A, Lee D, Deutsch G, et al. Oral manifestations as the first presenting sign of Crohn's disease in a pediatric patient. J Clin Exp Dent 2017;9(7):e934–8.

35. Pittock S, Drumm B, Fleming P, et al. The oral cavity in Crohn's disease. J Pediatr 2001;138(5):767–71.

36. Cizenski JD, Michel P, Watson IT, et al. Spectrum of orocutaneous disease associations: Immune-mediated conditions. J Am Acad Dermatol 2017; 77(5):795–806.

37. Jukema JB, Brandse JF, De Boer NK. Successful Treatment of Oral Crohn's Disease by Ustekinumab. Inflamm Bowel Dis 2020. https://doi.org/10.1093/ ibd/izz321.

38. Lazzerini M, Martelossi S, Cont G, et al. Orofacial granulomatosis in children: think about Crohn's disease. Dig Liver Dis 2015;47(4):338–41.

39. Grunewald J, Grutter JC, Arkema EV, et al. Sarcoidosis. Nat Rev Dis Primers 2019;5(1):45.

40. Motswaledi MH, Khammissa RAG, Jadwat Y, et al. Oral sarcoidosis: a case report and review of the literature. Aust Dent J 2014;59:389–94.

41. Suresh L, Radfar L. Oral sarcoidosis: a review of literature. Oral Dis 2005;11:138–45.

42. Poate TWJ, Sharma R, Moutasim KA, et al. Orofacial presentations of sarcoidosis – a case series and review of the literature. Br Dent J 2008;205(8):437–42.

43. Wanat KA, Rosenbach M. A practical approach to cutaneous sarcoidosis. Am J Clin Dermatol 2014; 15(4):283–97.

44. Al-Hamad A, Porter S, Fedele S. Orofacial Granulomatosis. Dermatol Clin 2015;33(3):433–46.

45. van der Waal RI, Schulten EA, van der Meij EH, et al. Cheilitis granulomatosa: overview of 13 patients with long-term follow-up–results of management. Int J Dermatol 2002;41(4):225–9.

46. Hullah EA, Escudier MP. The mouth in inflammatory bowel disease and aspects of orofacial granulomatosis. Periodontol 2000 2019;80(1):61–76.

47. Miest R, Bruce A, Rogers RS. Orofacial granulomatosis. Clin Dermatol 2016;34(4):505–13.

48. Sabet-Peyman EJ, Woodward JA. A case series of patients diagnosed with orofacial granulomatosis presenting primarily with dense infiltrates and severe periorbital edema. Ophthal Plast Reconstr Surg 2014;30(6):e151–5.

49. Du J, Zhang Y, Liu D, et al. Hodgkin's lymphoma with marked granulomatous reaction: a diagnostic pitfall. Int J Clin Exp Pathol 2019;12(7):2772–4.

50. Goto H, Sugita K, Shindo M, et al. Granuloma formation clinically presenting as erythroderma in a patient with peripheral T-cell lymphoma. Eur J Dermatol 2019;29(3):324–6.

51. Geetha D, Jefferson JA. ANCA-Associated Vasculitis: Core Curriculum 2020. Am J Kidney Dis 2020; 75(1):124–37.

52. Msallem B, Bassetti S, Matter MS, et al. Strawberry gingivitis: Challenges in the diagnosis of granulomatosis with polyangiitis on gingival specimens. Oral Surg Oral Med Oral Pathol Oral Radiol 2019; 128(6):e202–7.

53. Jariwala M, Laxer RM. Childhood GPA, EGPA, and MPA. Clin Immunol 2019;211:108325.

54. Stewart C, Cohen D, Bhattacharyya I, et al. Oral manifestations of Wegener's granulomatosis: a report of three cases and a literature review. J Am Dent Assoc 2007;138(3):338–48.

55. Thompson G, Benwell N, Hollingsworth P, et al. Two cases of granulomatosis polyangiitis presenting with Strawberry gingivitis and a review of the literature. Semin Arthritis Rheum 2018;47(4):520–3.

Acute Oral Lesions

Katherine France, DMD, MBE[a],*, Alessandro Villa, DDS, PhD, MPH[b]

KEYWORDS

- Oral lesions • Ulcers • Mucosal disease • Infectious diseases • Mouth sores

KEY POINTS

- A variety of acute oral lesions may be encountered in the practice of dermatology, many of which are common in the general population across demographic categories.
- Oral lesions arise from a wide variety of causes including infectious and autoimmune conditions, trauma, and secondary effects of systemic diseases and medications.
- Careful assessment of these lesions may allow for clinical diagnosis, appropriate treatment, or referral to provide effective and high-quality care.
- Many acute oral lesions are self-limiting in nature and do not require diagnostic testing or dedicated management.

BRIEF INTRODUCTION

Acute oral mucosal lesions are common and may be encountered in the general practice of dermatology.[1–4] Oral lesions may be single or multiple and may arise secondary to infectious, immunologic, congenital, reactive, or idiopathic causes. Several acute oral conditions may represent manifestations of a systemic disease or may arise secondary to medication use. As such, a thorough medical and drug history is important for accurate diagnosis and management. Patients should be queried on the duration (eg, length of time present), frequency, and symptoms (eg, pain, burning, sensitivity) associated with the oral condition. A referral to an appropriate specialist may be needed for further evaluation and treatment.

IMMUNE-MEDIATED CONDITIONS
Recurrent Aphthous Stomatitis and Aphthous-Like Ulcers

Recurrent aphthous stomatitis (RAS), also called canker sores, is a common immune-mediated condition present in up to 20% of the population.[5] RAS typically manifests in childhood or adolescence and becomes less frequent in adulthood (>40 year old).[5,6] The frequency of RAS is variable, but patients often experience oral ulcers either a few times a year or on a monthly basis. Some women may develop small oral ulcerations (aphthae) a few days before the menstrual cycle. The ulcerations are nondescript and vary in size and depth.

The true pathobiology of RAS has not been fully elucidated and many cases remain idiopathic.[7] For some patients, triggering factors have been identified including genetics, stress, hormonal changes, immunologic factors, local trauma, smoking cessation, some hypersensitivity reactions, and vitamin B_{12} and D deficiency.[7,8] Of note, many systemic diseases, including anemia and gastrointestinal conditions, may be accompanied by aphthous-like ulcers and patients should be carefully evaluated for possible concomitant systemic conditions.

Aphthous ulcers present as round shallow lesions covered by a yellowish fibrin layer with surrounding erythema (Fig. 1). RAS usually affects the nonkeratinized mucosa (mostly the labial and buccal mucosae) and resolves with no scarring between episodes. One exception is major RAS (discussed later), which may affect the keratinized

[a] Department of Oral Medicine, University of Pennsylvania School of Dental Medicine, 240 South 40th Street, Philadelphia, PA 19104, USA; [b] Department of Orofacial Sciences, University of California San Francisco, 513 Parnassus Avenue, Suite 512A, San Francisco, CA 94143, USA
* Corresponding author.
E-mail address: kfrance@upenn.edu

Dermatol Clin 38 (2020) 441–450
https://doi.org/10.1016/j.det.2020.05.005

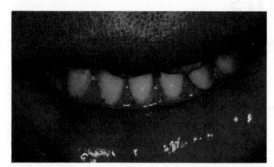

Fig. 1. Aphthous ulcer of the lower lip mucosa.

mucosa, such as the dorsal tongue, attached gingiva, or hard palatal mucosa. RAS is classified into three forms: (1) minor, (2) major, and (3) herpetiform. Ulceration related to systemic disease is often referred to as aphthous-like ulcers. Minor RAS is the most common form; minor ulcers are usually less than 1 cm in diameter and may be single or multiple.[7] Major aphthous ulcers are greater than 1.0 cm in diameter, deep, and painful. In herpetiform aphthous stomatitis, patients present with multiple small ulcers that resemble a herpes simplex virus (HSV) infection (discussed later). These usually heal within 7 to 10 days. Patients with severe aphthous stomatitis are almost never ulcer free, and as a result present with persistent oral pain, malnutrition, and weight loss. A biopsy is usually not indicated unless another condition or systemic cause is suspected (eg, a vesiculobullous disease) and when performed, histology shows an ulcer with markers of acute and chronic inflammation.

Regardless of the cause (idiopathic vs manifestation of a systemic disease), management goals are to reduce frequency and severity of the outbreaks and to control pain. Management for minor cases involves the use of over-the-counter local anesthetics (eg, benzocaine 10%), or mucoadhesive agents, such as polyvinylpyrrolidone sodium hyaluronate and methylcellulose paste. When necessary, management of RAS can include topical corticosteroids (eg, triamcinolone 0.1%, dexamethasone elixir 0.5 mg/5 mL) and/or other immunosuppressants. Patients with large lesions (>1 cm) may benefit from intralesional steroid therapy with triamcinolone (1 mg/cm^3 of ulcer). Systemic therapy with prednisone may be necessary to control severe cases until other agents are used. Other systemic agents proposed for recalcitrant cases include pentoxifylline, dapsone, colchicine, azathioprine, or thalidomide.[9]

Aphthous-like lesions have also been associated with several systemic conditions where the ulcers do not resolve in the typical 1 to 2 weeks. Aphthous-like ulcers may develop in patients with vitamins B_1, B_2, B_6, or B_{12} or folic acid and iron deficiency.[10,11] A blood test is recommended to confirm the cause of the ulcers if hematologic deficiencies are suspected.

Another condition associated with aphthous ulcers is periodic fever syndrome (periodic fever, aphthae, pharyngitis, adenopathy) in young patients (10–20 years of age).[12]

Celiac disease (celiac sprue, gluten-sensitive enteropathy) is an autoimmune disorder of the small intestine caused by a hypersensitivity reaction to gliadin, a gluten protein.[13] Aphthous-like ulcers may develop in 3% to 61% of patients with celiac.[14] Serologic testing is recommended in patients with oral ulcerations who also exhibit gastrointestinal symptoms (eg, malabsorption, abdominal pain, recurrent diarrhea, or constipation). IgA anti–tissue transglutaminase antibody is the preferred test for detection of celiac disease in adults.[15] In addition, total IgA levels and antigliadin antibody may be also checked.[16] Signs and symptoms, including oral ulcers, typically improve with a gluten-free diet. Hypersensitivities to other foods, including chocolate or eggs, may also cause aphthous ulcers.

Oral aphthous-like ulcers may also be present in patients affected by ulcerative colitis and Crohn disease. Associated signs and symptoms include fever, fatigue, diarrhea, abdominal pain and cramping, weight loss, and anemia.[17,18] Patients with ulcerative colitis may present with oral ulcerations (**Fig. 2**) and pyostomatitis vegetans (**Fig. 3**), a condition characterized by oral pustular and ulcerative eruptions. These pustules often coalesce and break down leaving superficial erosions. Oral aphthous ulcers in Crohn disease typically manifest with a linear appearance, especially if affecting the vestibular area.[19] These ulcers may also have indurated borders and histologic features portending their granulomatous nature.[20] Patients may also develop lip swelling, edema of the face, gingiva and oral mucosae with a characteristic cobblestone appearance, and angular cheilitis (**Fig. 4**).

Management of inflammatory bowel diseases involves an induction and maintenance regimen. Commonly used agents include corticosteroids, immunosuppressants (thiopurines [azathioprine and mercaptopurine] and methotrexate), biologic agents (anti–tumor necrosis factor [adalimumab, infliximab, and certolizumab pegol]), and antiadhesion molecules (vedolizumab).[21] Specific cases (eg, stricture or penetrating lesions) may require surgical intervention. Of note, patients undergoing ileectomy may develop aphthous-like ulcers from vitamin B_{12} deficiency secondary to malabsorption.[22]

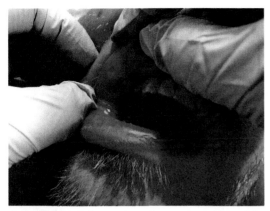

Fig. 2. Two aphthous ulcerations presenting on the upper labial mucosa in a patient with ulcerative colitis. (*Courtesy of* Thomas P. Sollecito, DMD, FDS RCSEd, Philadelphia, PA.)

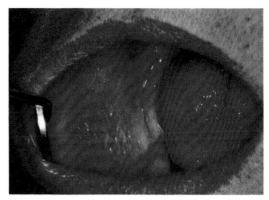

Fig. 4. Right buccal mucosa with a characteristic cobblestone appearance in a patient affected by Crohn disease.

Although the prevalence of oral conditions in patients with human immunodeficiency virus/acquired immunodeficiency syndrome (HIV/AIDS) has decreased after the advent of antiretroviral therapy, patients living with HIV/AIDS may still present with major aphthous-like oral ulcers that affect nonkeratinized and keratinized mucosa.[23] A biopsy is needed in these patients to rule out other diseases, such as infectious conditions (eg, deep fungal infections). The ulcers usually resolve once the underlying disease is effectively managed and concomitant topical and/or systemic steroid therapy can be used adjunctively.

Erythema Multiforme

Erythema multiforme (EM) is a self-limiting mucocutaneous disease with acute onset showing association with HLA-DRw53, DQw3, and Aw33 antigens.[24] Most cases occur between the second and fourth decades of life with a slight male predominance.[25] Several factors have been linked with EM including use of certain medications (eg, anticonvulsants, nonsteroidal anti-inflammatory drugs, and sulfonamides), infections (mostly a hypersensitivity reaction to a recent HSV infection, asymptomatic or subclinical HSV reactivation, or *Mycoplasma pneumoniae*), and menstruation.[26,27] Malaise, headache, fever, and sore throat may develop a few days to 1 to 2 weeks before the onset of lesions. Lesions in the oral cavity are characterized by ulcerations, pain, and crusted ulcerated lips. Cutaneous lesions appear in a symmetric distribution as erythematous and raised papules with a target or bull's eye appearance and typically affect the extensor surfaces of the acral extremities.[25] The ocular and genital mucosa can also be affected. Lesions typically last 2 to 4 weeks and heal without scarring.

Two forms of EM are recognized: minor and major. EM major affects the skin and at least one mucosal site or may show extensive involvement of a single mucosal site.[28] EM minor is mostly cutaneous with less than 10% of skin surface affected and little to no mucosal involvement, although a few cases may affect the mouth only.[29] The diagnosis is usually made based on clinical findings and biopsy may be helpful as confirmation or when the clinical presentation is ambiguous. An oral culture (viral polymerase chain reaction) may be obtained to rule out HSV infection. In cases of possible *M pneumoniae* infection, a chest radiograph, polymerase chain reaction testing of throat swabs, and serologic tests are recommended.[29] Management of EM is with topical and systemic analgesics and skin wound care; severe cases of mucosal EM may require hospital-based comfort measures.[30] Systemic glucocorticoids are frequently prescribed to shorten the course of the disease and decrease the severity of symptoms.

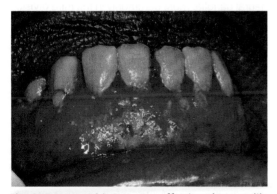

Fig. 3. Pyostomatitis vegetans affecting the mandibular gingiva. (*Courtesy of* Thomas P. Sollecito, DMD, FDS RCSEd, Philadelphia, PA.)

Stevens-Johnson syndrome (SJS) and toxic epidermal necrolysis (TEN) are severe mucocutaneous reactions and are considered separate entities from EM. Most cases are triggered by certain drugs (eg, allopurinol, imidazole antifungals, nevirapine, anticonvulsants, sulfonamides, or nonsteroidal anti-inflammatory drugs).[31] HLA-B*15:02 is a genetic marker associated with carbamazepine-induced SJS.[32] The Food and Drug Administration suggests screening Asian and South Asian patients for HLA-B*15:02 if carbamazepine use is under consideration because this allele is seen in high frequency in many Asian populations.[33] Similarly to EM major, patients with SJS and TEN present with large mucosal ulcerations and hemorrhagic lip crusting. Cutaneous erosions and blistering are always present. Cutaneous detachment affects less than 10% of skin of the body surface in SJS, greater than 30% in TEN, and 10% to 30% in patients with SJS/TEN overlap. Supportive care is the mainstay of treatment. The use of intravenous immunoglobulin remains controversial. Cyclosporine may be used as adjunct therapy.[34]

INFECTIOUS CONDITIONS
Herpetic Gingivostomatitis, Recurrent Herpes Simplex Virus Infections

Herpetic gingivostomatitis occurs as a manifestation of initial infection with HSV-1 or HSV-2. In approximately 20% to 30% of patients, primary infection with either of these viruses causes painful oral ulcerations lasting 7 to 10 days.[35] Approximately 90% of cases are caused by HSV-1,[36] whereas HSV-2 more commonly affects the genital mucosa and can cause a similar clinical appearance. Although most US adults have been exposed to HSV-1, the primary infection is subclinical in most patients.[37] The virus gains access to the host through exposure to mucosal secretions of an infected individual, commonly oral or nasal. Primary herpetic gingivostomatitis occurs most commonly up to age 6 and shows another peak of incidence in the late second decade, as initiation of sexual activity exposes some persons not previously infected.[36]

Herpetic gingivostomatitis manifests as painful clusters of 1- to 5-mm ulcers on the nonkeratinized and keratinized oral mucosa, enlargement of gingiva, and mucosal hemorrhage (**Fig. 5**). Lesions begin as vesicles and rupture to form multiple bilateral ulcerations. These can be asymptomatic but are often acutely painful and can interfere with oral intake. Before oral lesions are visible, and throughout the self-limiting course of the condition, patients often experience fever, malaise,

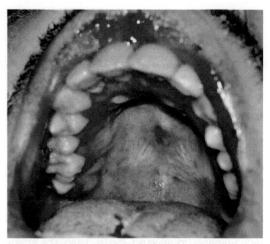

Fig. 5. Herpetic gingivostomatitis affecting the upper lip, hard palate, and anterior tongue.

and cervical lymphadenopathy.[38] Diagnosis of the condition is most commonly reached clinically and may be aided by a history of recent contact with an infected host. When necessary, viral testing of a lesion can confirm the diagnosis.[39] Although painful and esthetically objectionable, these lesions heal without scarring.

Treatment of herpetic gingivostomatitis is primarily palliative, consisting of topical and systemic pain control (2% viscous lidocaine rinses, combination rinses [ie, anesthetic, antihistamine, antacid], oral acetaminophen).[40] Systemic treatment of herpetic gingivostomatitis is usually not warranted, but systemic antivirals can shorten the course of the disease if started in the first 3 days.[35] Occasionally, pain and poor intake may require hospitalization for supportive care.[41] Rarely, patients develop serious or life-threatening complications, such as herpes simplex encephalitis.[36]

After initial infection, the herpes virus resides in neural ganglia, most commonly in the third division (V3) root of the trigeminal nerve, where physical or emotional stress can cause reactivation.[37] Recurrent herpes infections occur in approximately 40% of patients.[37] Reactivation most commonly manifests clinically as recurrent herpes labialis (cold sores), a coalescence of vesicles on the outer labial surface at the vermilion border. These lesions shed viral particles, particularly during the early prodrome, and patients should exercise caution in contact with persons who may not carry the virus.[42] Recurrent HSV infections can also manifest intraorally as a gingivostomatitis as described previously. In immunocompetent individuals, recurrent intraoral herpes appears as clustered vesicles that evolve into ulcerations on attached gingiva, commonly in the palate. These recurrences are minimally painful, asymptomatic, and heal within 10 days. Recurrent intraoral herpes is most common, however, in immunosuppressed individuals. In this population, clusters of vesicles occur more commonly on unattached tissue, may be more widespread, and present with more significant pain and difficulty eating and speaking.[43] Treatment of reactivations is primarily symptomatic (**Table 1**). Length of flare may be decreased by using topical or systemic agents if started within 48 to 72 hours.[37,44]

Varicella Zoster Virus

Varicella zoster virus (VZV) is also a member of the human herpesvirus family (HHV-3) and can manifest similarly to HSV-1 and HSV-2 during acute and recurrent infections. Primary varicella infection (chickenpox) may include bilateral small oral vesicles that rupture into shallow but widespread painful ulcerations.[44] These oral lesions are present in most severe cases of chickenpox, and are more rare in mild to moderate cases.[45] Oral lesions can often be managed with hydration and analgesics but patients with severe or widespread lesions may require hospitalization for supportive care.

As with HSV-1 and HSV-2, VZV remains latent in neural ganglia and can be reactivated. Reactivation frequency increases with age and is seen more frequently in immunocompromised patients.[46] The recurrent infection is known as herpes zoster (shingles). Herpes zoster manifests as unilateral coalescing vesicles in following the distribution of a nerve. Zoster can occur in any area of the body and affects the trigeminal nerve in about 15% of cases. Trigeminal herpes zoster most commonly affects the ophthalmic branch (V1) and can rarely cause intraoral manifestations in cases affecting the mandibular branch (V3).[35,37] Intraoral lesions become apparent after

Table 1
Topical and systemic agents to manage HSV infections

Topical Agents	Instructions
Acyclovir 5% ointment Penciclovir 1% ointment Docosanol 10%	Apply to lesions every 2 h for 7 d
Systemic Agents	
Acyclovir 400 mg and 800 mg tablet	Primary HSV infection a. 800 mg 2–5 times/d for 7–10 d b. 400 mg 3 times/d for 7–10 d Recurrent HSV infection a. 400 mg 3 times/d for 5 d b. 800 mg twice/day for 5 d
Valacyclovir 500 mg and 1000 mg caplet	Primary HSV infection 1 g twice/day for 7–10 d Recurrent HSV infection 500 mg twice daily for 3 d Labial HSV infection 2 g at first sign of recurrence, then 2 g 12 h later Prophylaxis (when precipitating event is known) 2 g twice on the day of the dental procedure or event, then 1 g twice the next day (up to 1–3 d after the event or procedure) Immunosuppressed individuals 1 g daily VZV infection 1 g 3 times/d for 7–14 d
Famciclovir 125 mg and 250 mg tablet	Primary HSV infection 250 mg 3 times/d for 7–10 d Recurrent HSV infection 125 mg twice/day for 5 d VZV infection 500 mg 3 times/d for 7–14 d

Abbreviation: VZV, varicella zoster virus.

a prodromal period of approximately 72 hours and affect keratinized and nonkeratinized mucosa.[47] Both varicella and zoster are diagnosed clinically, and the diagnosis is confirmed with viral polymerase chain reaction or biopsy.[47] A zoster flare may also be treated with antivirals (see **Table 1**).[44] Herpes zoster flares, including in the oral cavity, may lead to postherpetic neuralgia, a potentially long-standing and recalcitrant pain condition. Postherpetic neuralgia consists of a continued sharp pain in the area of a previous zoster flare after the healing of viral lesions. Postherpetic neuralgia is estimated to occur in about 10% of cases but may be lower in patients treated appropriately during flares. A childhood vaccine against VZV and a subunit vaccine specifically targeting zoster also exist and may decrease frequency and severity of flares.[47]

Coxsackievirus

Coxsackievirus infection presents two variations: hand-foot-and-mouth disease (HFMD) and herpangina. HFMD is most commonly caused by coxsackievirus A16 and enterovirus 17.[48] Occasionally seen in adults, it most commonly manifests in children younger than age 5 as a combination of systemic signs including fever and malaise; oral ulcerations covering the labial, buccal, and palatal mucosa; and vesicular skin eruptions on the palms and soles.[49] In adults, in children younger than 2 years of age, and when caused by more rare serotypes, HFMD is more likely to lead to severe disease and complications, such as aseptic meningitis and encephalitis.[49] Some cases of HFMD may not show all classical components. Herpangina is a more localized manifestation limited to fever and multiple small coalescent ulcers on the soft palatal mucosa and tonsillar pillars.[50]

HFMD is self-limiting and usually lasts 7 to 10 days.[50] Most patients only require supportive care including hydration and pain management.[49] In severe cases, more of the body surface or internal organs may become infected and patients may require systemic treatment. Intravenous immunoglobulin has been used successfully, and interferon alpha-1b may decrease the length and severity of the infection, including hastening the healing of oral lesions.[49,51]

OTHER ULCERS
Ulcerations in Cyclic Neutropenia

Cyclic neutropenia is a rare genetic disease caused by mutations in the neutrophil elastase gene ELANE, causing patients to experience a severe decrease in neutrophils (absolute neutrophil count $<0.2 \times 10^9$/L) followed by recovery approximately every 21 days.[52,53] This disease causes many clinical manifestations and systemic complications, including oral ulcerations during the neutrophil nadir in 97% of patients.[54] At times, oral ulcerations are the presenting sign of the disease, particularly when they occur at a young age in concert with fever and infection. Ulcerations are often deep and painful, can occur on all types of oral mucosa, and tend to manifest regularly, even as systemic signs of nadir, such as fever and infections, decrease with age.[55] Patients with cyclic neutropenia are occasionally treated with granulocyte colony–stimulating factor multiple times weekly.[55,56] Enforcement of good oral hygiene and routine periodontal maintenance can also minimize the burden of oral disease in this population.[57]

Traumatic Ulcers

Ulcers may also arise after thermal, mechanical, or chemical trauma. Thermal insults range from hot food and drink to electric burns. Mechanical trauma may occur because of single or multiple insults from teeth or external sources. Chemical burns have been reported from a wide variety of sources including aspirin and other medications, topical or systemic exposure to acids including sulfuric acid and hydrogen peroxide, dental materials including sodium hypochlorite, recreational drugs, and foods including garlic.[58,59] Traumatic ulcers can occur in any area of the oral mucosa, represent a wide range of sizes, and are most effectively treated with removal of the causative agent. This may include changing habits, adjusting dental prostheses, or smoothing sharp tooth cusps. Once an agent is removed, the patient should be monitored for healing within 2 to 4 weeks.

If traumatic ulcers do not heal with removal of the suspected cause, biopsy is warranted to rule out malignancy or other underlying disease.[43] Traumatic ulceration of the oral mucosa often demonstrates coagulation necrosis on biopsy or a mixed infiltrate of lymphocytes and histiocytes with marked eosinophilia, consistent with an entity known as traumatic ulcerative granuloma with stromal eosinophilia (TUGSE).[60] TUGSE is most common in patients in their 40s to 60s, particularly denture-wearers, with equal sex prevalence. TUGSE is clinically remarkable as a persistent, rapidly expansile ulcer with keratotic rims that raises concern for malignancy because of its size and firm elevated borders, but represents a benign deep traumatic ulcer often caused by chronic irritation.[61] TUGSE often heal independently after biopsy. Ulcers proven to be benign on biopsy are treated with topical, intralesional, and systemic corticosteroids as needed to supplement healing.[62,63]

Necrotizing Sialometaplasia

Necrotizing sialometaplasia is a benign, self-limiting reaction to ischemia by the minor or occasionally major salivary glands (**Fig. 6**). Once the diagnosis is properly established, the lesion may be monitored and does not require additional treatment. However, given the clinical similarity to certain malignant entities (eg, squamous cell carcinoma and mucoepidermoid carcinoma), incisional biopsy is essential for diagnosis. Necrotizing sialometaplasia manifests most commonly on the hard palatal mucosa, followed by the soft palate, floor of mouth, and lateral tongue.[64] The lesion often presents as a unilateral, painful, erythematous, well-defined raised ulceration of 1 cm or more diameter, which may expose, but does not involve, the underlying bone.[65] The ulcerations are often deep and may exhibit desquamation.[66] The area of the lesion may or may not correspond to an area of trauma including from dental procedures (eg, greater palatine anesthetic block), dentures, or previous surgery. Cases have also been reported to correlate with other causes of ischemia, including anorexia and bulimia nervosa, smoking, alcohol use, Raynaud phenomenon, Buerger disease (thromboangiitis obliterans), and topical medications including nonsteroidal anti-inflammatory drugs, all of which are hypothesized to cause a localized vasculitis.[67,68] Once diagnosed, no active treatment is required. Local protective devices may be used to prevent further trauma.[69]

OTHER ACUTE ORAL LESIONS
Mucoceles

Mucoceles are the clinical manifestation of mucous extravasation from the minor salivary glands.

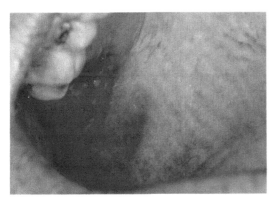

Fig. 6. Necrotizing sialometaplasia of the posterior right palatal mucosa.

These benign lesions occur secondary to trauma or because of mucous build up in the glands. They can occur in any mucosal surface containing minor salivary glands but are most common on the lower lip, floor of the mouth, and buccal mucosa.[70] Mucoceles are the most common salivary gland pathology in the oral cavity.[70] They occur most commonly in teenage and young adult patients but can present at any age.[71]

Mucoceles are less than 1 cm in size and tend to be single, round, well-circumscribed lesions that can appear clear, red, or blue in color depending on the extent of trauma to the surrounding mucosal structures. Although they tend to be asymptomatic, larger lesions can interfere with function and present esthetic concerns. Mucoceles often require excision, and clinicians must carefully excise the damaged minor salivary glands and any surrounding affected tissue to minimize the chance of recurrence. Recurrence can still occur, however, and new mucoceles can form after new trauma in adjacent areas. In addition to excision, mucoceles are treated using marsupialization, local infiltration of corticosteroid, laser excision, or cryotherapy.[72]

SUMMARY

Acute oral ulcerations may be associated with a variety of pathophysiologic mechanisms and clinical disorders. The evaluation of the patient presenting with an oral ulceration involves a careful medical and medication history accompanied by a thorough intraoral and extraoral examination. Some cases may require a biopsy and histopathologic examination to confirm the initial diagnosis. Treatment of acute oral lesions requires a multidisciplinary approach, especially if they are secondary to a systemic condition.

DISCLOSURE

The authors have nothing to disclose.

REFERENCES

1. Axéll T. A prevalence study of oral mucosal lesions in an adult Swedish population. Odontol Revy Suppl 1976;36:1–103.
2. Carrard V, Haas A, Rados P, et al. Prevalence and risk indicators of oral mucosal lesions in an urban population from South Brazil. Oral Dis 2011;17(2):171–9.
3. García-Pola Vallejo MJ, Martínez Díaz-Canel AI, García Martín JM, et al. Risk factors for oral soft tissue lesions in an adult Spanish population. Community Dent Oral Epidemiol 2002;30(4):277–85.

4. Pentenero M, Broccoletti R, Carbone M, et al. The prevalence of oral mucosal lesions in adults from the Turin area. Oral Dis 2008;14(4):356–66.

5. Scully C. Clinical practice. Aphthous ulceration. N Engl J Med 2006;355(2):165–72.

6. Ship JA, Chavez EM, Doerr PA, et al. Recurrent aphthous stomatitis. Quintessence Int 2000;31(2): 95–112.

7. Baccaglini L, Lalla RV, Bruce AJ, et al. Urban legends: recurrent aphthous stomatitis. Oral Dis 2011; 17(8):755–70.

8. Al-Maweri SA, Halboub E, Al-Sufyani G, et al. Is vitamin D deficiency a risk factor for recurrent aphthous stomatitis? A systematic review and meta-analysis. Oral Dis 2019. https://doi.org/10.1111/odi.13189.

9. Hello M, Barbarot S, Bastuji-Garin S, et al. Use of thalidomide for severe recurrent aphthous stomatitis: a multicenter cohort analysis. Medicine (Baltimore) 2010;89(3):176–82.

10. Kozlak ST, Walsh SJ, Lalla RV. Reduced dietary intake of vitamin B12 and folate in patients with recurrent aphthous stomatitis. J Oral Pathol Med 2010;39(5):420–3.

11. Lalla RV, Choquette LE, Feinn RS, et al. Multivitamin therapy for recurrent aphthous stomatitis: a randomized, double-masked, placebo-controlled trial. J Am Dent Assoc 2012;143(4):370–6.

12. Wekell P, Karlsson A, Berg S, et al. Review of auto-inflammatory diseases, with a special focus on periodic fever, aphthous stomatitis, pharyngitis and cervical adenitis syndrome. Acta Paediatr 2016; 105(10):1140–51.

13. Houlston RS, Tomlinson IP, Ford D, et al. Linkage analysis of candidate regions for coeliac disease genes. Hum Mol Genet 1997;6(8):1335–9.

14. Scully C, Hodgson T. Recurrent oral ulceration: aphthous-like ulcers in periodic syndromes. Oral Surg Oral Med Oral Pathol Oral Radiol Endod 2008;106(6):845–52.

15. Barker JM, Liu E. Celiac disease: pathophysiology, clinical manifestations, and associated autoimmune conditions. Adv Pediatr 2008;55:349–65.

16. Pelkowski TD, Viera AJ. Celiac disease: diagnosis and management. Am Fam Physician 2014;89(2): 99–105.

17. Ungaro R, Mehandru S, Allen PB, et al. Ulcerative colitis. Lancet 2017;389(10080):1756–70.

18. Torres J, Mehandru S, Colombel JF, et al. Crohn's disease. Lancet 2017;389(10080):1741–55.

19. Baumgart DC, Sandborn WJ. Crohn's disease. Lancet 2012;380(9853):1590–605.

20. Akintoye SO, Greenberg MS. Recurrent aphthous stomatitis. Dent Clin North Am 2014;58(2):281–97.

21. Baumgart DC, Sandborn WJ. Inflammatory bowel disease: clinical aspects and established and evolving therapies. Lancet 2007;369(9573): 1641–57.

22. Villa A, Woo SB. Oral manifestations of systemic diseases. In: Michael Glick, editor. The oral-systemic health connection: a guide to patient care. 2nd edition. Batavia, Illinois: Quintessence Symposium; 2018. p. 242–70.

23. Patton LL. Oral lesions associated with human immunodeficiency virus disease. Dent Clin North Am 2013;57(4):673–98.

24. Kampgen E, Burg G, Wank R. Association of herpes simplex virus-induced erythema multiforme with the human leukocyte antigen DQw3. Arch Dermatol 1988;124(9):1372–5.

25. Huff JC, Weston WL, Tonnesen MG. Erythema multiforme: a critical review of characteristics, diagnostic criteria, and causes. J Am Acad Dermatol 1983;8(6): 763–5.

26. Williams PM, Conklin RJ. Erythema multiforme: a review and contrast from Stevens-Johnson syndrome/toxic epidermal necrolysis. Dent Clin North Am 2005;49(1):67–76, viii.

27. Leaute-Labreze C, Lamireau T, Chawki D, et al. Diagnosis, classification, and management of erythema multiforme and Stevens-Johnson syndrome. Arch Dis Child 2000;83(4):347–52.

28. Lamoreux MR, Sternbach MR, Hsu WT. Erythema multiforme. Am Fam Physician 2006;74(11):1883–8.

29. Sokumbi O, Wetter DA. Clinical features, diagnosis, and treatment of erythema multiforme: a review for the practicing dermatologist. Int J Dermatol 2012; 51(8):889–902.

30. Ayangco L, Rogers RS 3rd. Oral manifestations of erythema multiforme. Dermatol Clin 2003;21(1): 195–205.

31. Stern RS, Divito SJ. Stevens-Johnson syndrome and toxic epidermal necrolysis: associations, outcomes, and pathobiology-thirty years of progress but still much to be done. J Invest Dermatol 2017;137(5):1004–8.

32. Chung WH, Hung SI, Hong HS, et al. Medical genetics: a marker for Stevens-Johnson syndrome. Nature 2004;428(6982):486.

33. Tangamornsuksan W, Chaiyakunapruk N, Somkrua R, et al. Relationship between the HLA-B*1502 allele and carbamazepine-induced Stevens-Johnson syndrome and toxic epidermal necrolysis: a systematic review and meta-analysis. JAMA Dermatol 2013;149(9):1025–32.

34. Khalili B, Bahna SL. Pathogenesis and recent therapeutic trends in Stevens-Johnson syndrome and toxic epidermal necrolysis. Ann Allergy Asthma Immunol 2006;97(3):272–80 [quiz: 281-273, 320].

35. Abdel-Naby Awad OG, Hamad A-MH. Honey can help in herpes simplex gingivostomatitis in children: prospective randomized double blind placebo controlled clinical trial. Am J Otolaryngol 2018; 39(6):759–63.

36. Goldman RD. Acyclovir for herpetic gingivostomatitis in children. Can Fam Physician 2016;62(5):403–4.

37. Hargitai IA. Painful oral lesions. Dent Clin North Am 2018;62(4):597–609.
38. Kolokotronis A, Doumas S. Herpes simplex virus infection, with particular reference to the progression and complications of primary herpetic gingivostomatitis. Clin Microbiol Infect 2006;12(3):202–11.
39. Mohan RP, Verma S, Singh U, et al. Acute primary herpetic gingivostomatitis. BMJ Case Rep 2013. https://doi.org/10.1136/bcr-2013-200074.
40. Faden H. Management of primary herpetic gingivostomatitis in young children. Pediatr Emerg Care 2006;22(4):268–9.
41. Allareddy V, Elangovan S. Characteristics of hospitalizations attributed to herpetic gingivostomatitis: analysis of nationwide inpatient sample. Oral Surg Oral Med Oral Pathol Oral Radiol 2014;117(4):471–6.
42. Ramdass P, Mullick S, Farber HF. Viral skin diseases. Prim Care 2015;42(4):517–67.
43. Fitzpatrick SG, Cohen DM, Clark AN. Ulcerated lesions of the oral mucosa: clinical and histologic review. Head Neck Pathol 2019;13(1):91–102.
44. Rosen T. Recurrent herpes labialis in adults: new tricks for an old dog. J Drugs Dermatol 2017;16(3):s49–53.
45. Kolokotronis A, Louloudaidis K, Fotiou G, et al. Oral manifestations of infections due to varicella zoster virus in otherwise healthy children. J Clin Pediatr Dent 2001;25(2):107–12.
46. El Hayderi L, Rubben A, Nikkels AF. The alphaherpesviridae in dermatology: varicella zoster virus. Hautarzt 2017;68(Suppl 1):S6–10.
47. Mangold AR, Torgerson RR, Rogers RS. Diseases of the tongue. Clin Dermatol 2016;34(4):458–69.
48. Nassef C, Ziemer C, Morrell DS. Hand-foot-and-mouth disease: a new look at a classic viral rash. Curr Opin Pediatr 2015;27(4):486–91.
49. Ventarola D, Bordone L, Silverberg N. Update on hand-foot-and-mouth disease. Clin Dermatol 2015;33(3):340–6.
50. Kimmis BD, Downing C, Tyring S. Hand-foot-and-mouth disease caused by coxsackievirus A6 on the rise. Cutis 2018;102(5):353–6.
51. Huang X, Zhang X, Wang F, et al. Clinical efficacy of therapy with recombinant human interferon alpha-1b in hand, foot, and mouth disease with enterovirus 71 infection. PLoS One 2016;11(2):e0148907.
52. Patil VH, Hugar SM, Balikai G, et al. Severe congenital cyclic neutropenia: a case report. Int J Appl Basic Med Res 2016;6(4):293–6.
53. Makaryan V, Zeidler C, Bolyard AA, et al. The diversity of mutations and clinical outcomes for ELANE-associated neutropenia. Curr Opin Hematol 2015;22(1):3–11.
54. Chen X, Peng W, Zhang Z, et al. ELANE gene mutation-induced cyclic neutropenia manifesting as recurrent fever with oral mucosal ulcer: a case report. Medicine (Baltimore) 2018;97(10):e0031.
55. Aota K, Kani K, Yamanoi T, et al. Management of tooth extraction in a patient with ELANE gene mutation-induced cyclic neutropenia: a case report. Medicine (Baltimore) 2019;98(39):e17372.
56. Dale DC, Bolyard A, Marrero T, et al. Long-term effects of G-CSF therapy in cyclic neutropenia. N Engl J Med 2017;377(23):2290–2.
57. Chen Y, Fang L, Yang X. Cyclic neutropenia presenting as recurrent oral ulcers and periodontitis. J Clin Pediatr Dent 2013;37(3):307–8.
58. Dayakar MM, Pai PG, Sooranagi PM, et al. Chemical burns of gingiva and its management. SRM J Res Dent Sci 2018;9(4):174–80.
59. Gilvetti C, Porter SR, Fedele S. Traumatic chemical oral ulceration: a case report and review of the literature. Br Dent J 2010;208(7):297–300.
60. Panta P, Sarode SC, Sarode GS, et al. Chronic traumatic ulcer of lateral tongue: an underestimated oral potentially malignant disorder? Oral Oncol 2018;85:101–2.
61. Butler JN, Kobayashi TT. Traumatic ulcerative granuloma with stromal eosinophilia: a malignant-appearing benign lesion. Cutis 2017;100(2):e28–31.
62. Kuriyama Y, Shimizu A, Toki S, et al. Two cases of chronic oral ulcers effectively treated with systemic corticosteroid therapy: circumoroficial plasmacytosis and traumatic ulcerative granuloma with stromal eosinophilia. J Dermatol 2019;46(1):48–51.
63. Fantozzi PJ, Treister N, Shekar R, et al. Intralesional triamcinolone acetonide therapy for inflammatory oral ulcers. Oral Surg Oral Med Oral Pathol Oral Radiol 2019;128(5):485–90.
64. Zhurakivska K, Maiorano E, Nocini R, et al. Necrotizing sialometaplasia can hide the presence of salivary gland tumors: a case series. Oral Dis 2019;25(4):1084–90.
65. Carlson DL. Necrotizing sialometaplasia: a practical approach to the diagnosis. Arch Pathol Lab Med 2009;133(5):692–8.
66. Kandula S, Manjunatha BS, Tayee P, et al. Bilateral necrotising sialometaplasia. BMJ Case Rep 2016. https://doi.org/10.1136/bcr-2015-211348.
67. Gatti A, Broccardo E, Poglio G, et al. Necrotizing sialometaplasia of the hard palate in a patient treated with topical nonsteroidal anti-inflammatory drug. Case Rep Dent 2016;2016:9545861.
68. Senapati S, Samal SC, Kumar R, et al. Necrotizing sialometaplasia: manifestation of a localized unclassified vasculitis. Indian J Pathol Microbiol 2016;59(2):232–4.
69. Brannon RB, Fowler CB, Hartman KS. Necrotizing sialometaplasia. A clinicopathologic study of sixty-nine cases and review of the literature. Oral Surg Oral Med Oral Pathol 1991;72(3):317–25.

70. Joseph BK, Ali MA, Dashti H, et al. Analysis of oral and maxillofacial pathology lesions over an 18-year period diagnosed at Kuwait University. J Investig Clin Dent 2019;10(4):e12432.

71. Yu Z, Seo B, Hussaini HM, et al. The relative frequency of paediatric oral and maxillofacial pathology in New Zealand: a 10-year review of a national specialist centre. Int J Paediatr Dent 2020;30(2):209–15.

72. Choi YJ, Byun JS, Choi JK, et al. Identification of predictive variables for the recurrence of oral mucocele. Med Oral Patol Oral Cir Bucal 2019;24(2): e231–5.

Chronic Oral Lesions

Alaa F. Bukhari, BDS, MS[a],*, Arwa M. Farag, BDS, DMSc[a,b],
Nathaniel S. Treister, DMD, DMSc[c]

KEYWORDS

• Oral cavity • Skin • Chronic lesions • Mucocutaneus disease • Multidisciplinary management

KEY POINTS

- Chronic oral lesions are frequently observed in patients with dermatologic diseases.
- Oral lesions can be the first clinical sign of various mucocutaneous diseases.
- A multidisciplinary approach involving oral medicine and dermatology plays an essential role in patient management.

INTRODUCTION

A wide variety of chronic mucosal lesions observed in the oral cavity may precede or simultaneously present with cutaneous manifestations of disease. Causal factors may be autoimmune/immune-mediated, reactive, genetic, or infectious. Early diagnosis and proper multidisciplinary management can help ensure optimal clinical outcomes and quality of life. This article summarizes various chronic oral lesions frequently encountered in dermatology clinics.

IMMUNE-MEDIATED AND AUTOIMMUNE DISORDERS
Oral Lichen Planus

Epidemiology
Lichen planus (LP) is a chronic, mucocutaneous, immune-mediated disease that primarily affects skin and oral mucosa.[1] Oral LP (OLP) tends to occur more in women between 30 and 60 years of age, with estimated prevalence ranges between 0.5% and 2.2%.[1,2]

Pathobiology
OLP is a T cell–mediated immune response targeting keratinocytes in the basal cell layer, resulting in keratinocytic apoptosis.[2] Activation of cluster of differentiation (CD) 8+ cells, release of tumor necrotic factor alpha, and degranulation of mast cells are some of the proposed mechanisms involved in its pathogenesis.[2] Factors observed to be associated with OLP include stress, hepatitis C, thyroid disease, and hypersensitivity reactions.[3,4]

Clinical manifestations
Although oral lesions may be the only presentation of the disease, extraoral involvement (eg, skin, genitalia, esophagus, larynx, or conjunctiva) is common.[1] OLP is classically characterized by bilateral, symmetric distribution of the lesions on buccal mucosa, tongue, and gingiva. The disease has several clinical presentations that include reticular, ulcerative (erosive), and atrophic (erythematous).[5] The reticular form is the most common form of the disease.[6,7] It consists of asymptomatic intersecting white fine lines, known as Wickham striae, on normal mucosa or an erythematous background.[7] Plaquelike lesions are less commonly observed and can be confused with oral leukoplakia.[7] Patients with erosive-type lesions present with symptomatic, ulcerative lesions surrounded by erythema and/or radiating reticulations (**Fig. 1**). Some patients present with desquamative gingivitis (DG), characterized by erythematous changes and erosions limited to the attached and marginal gingiva (**Fig. 2**); this

a Department of Oral Diagnostic Sciences, Division of Oral Medicine, King Abdulaziz University, Faculty of Dentistry, Jeddah 21589, Saudi Arabia; b Department of Diagnostic Sciences, Division of Oral Medicine, Tufts University School of Dental Medicine, 1 Kneeland Street, Boston, MA 02111, USA; c Division of Oral and Maxillofacial Surgery, Oral Medicine and Dentistry, Brigham and Women's Hospital, 1620 Tremont Street, Boston, MA 02115, USA
* Corresponding author.
E-mail address: afnukhari@kau.edu.sa

Dermatol Clin 38 (2020) 451–466
https://doi.org/10.1016/j.det.2020.05.006

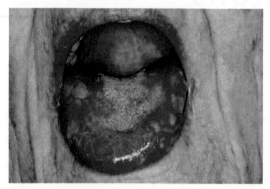

Fig. 1. Oral lichen planus of the right and left side of the tongue dorsum with prominent ulceration, reticulation, and erythema.

can be also seen in other vesiculobullous lesions such pemphigus vulgaris (PV), and mucous membrane pemphigoid (MMP).[8] Oral lesions occur in nearly 60% of the patients with cutaneous LP, whereas 15% of patients with oral lesions can develop cutaneous lesions.[8] Cutaneous lichen planus most commonly affects flexors of the extremities and presents bilaterally as purple, polygonal, pruritic papules or plaques covered by white striae.[9]

Diagnosis

Diagnosis of the reticular type is based on clinical characteristics. In most instances, erosive and plaquelike LP require tissue biopsy to confirm diagnosis. For DG, biopsy specimens should be submitted for routine histopathology and immunofluorescence studies to differentiate OLP from other vesiculobullous lesions such as PV and MMP.[2]

Histopathology

Histopathologic features of perilesional tissue include liquefactive degeneration of the basal cell

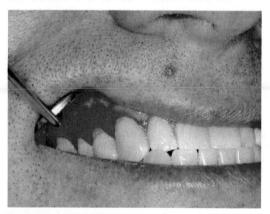

Fig. 2. Oral lichen planus presenting as desquamative gingivitis.

layer and bandlike lymphocytic infiltrate in the superficial layer of connective tissue.[3] Other microscopic features, such as hyperkeratosis, acanthosis, saw-toothed rete ridges, and cytoid (Civatte) bodies, can be seen.[3] Direct immunofluorescence (DIF) shows deposition of fibrinogen in a shaggy pattern along the basement membrane zone (BMZ).[3,8]

Management

Patients with asymptomatic disease do not require treatment other than periodic monitoring.[3] Symptomatic cases can be managed according to the severity and the extent of the disease. Off-label use of topical corticosteroids is considered the first-line therapy.[3] Localized lesions can be treated by applying a high-potency (eg, fluocinonide) or ultrapotency (eg, clobetasol) topical steroid gel on the lesions, whereas diffuse lesions are best managed by using a steroid oral rinse such as dexamethasone.[3] For patients with DG, topical steroid gel can be placed on custom-made occlusal trays to cover the affected areas of the gingiva.[6] Intralesional injections of triamcinolone acetonide (10–40 mg/mL) are used, in which injection of 0.1 mL/cm^3 is recommended for localized large ulcerations that do not respond to topical steroids.[1,3] Topical tacrolimus, a calcineurin inhibitor, can be used in the form of ointment 0.1% when topical corticosteroids are ineffective or contraindicated (**Table 1**).[3] Prophylactic antifungal therapy is considered in cases with prolonged use of corticosteroids or in patients with previous history of oral candidiasis. Sugar content of antifungal therapy must be taken into consideration in patients with salivary gland dysfunction.[1] Regular dental visits and topical fluoride application can help to reduce caries risk associated with xerostomia.[1] In refractory or severe oral cases, a short course of systemic prednisone (0.5–1 mg/kg/d) can be prescribed.[1] Systemic steroid-sparing agents, such as hydroxychloroquine, azathioprine, mycophenolate mofetil, and cyclosporine, can also be used.[3] Malignant transformation of OLP occurs in approximately 1% of cases.[1,10] Therefore, a long-term follow-up at least annually is necessary, with more frequent follow-up visits required for symptomatic lesions.[2,8]

Pemphigus Vulgaris

Epidemiology

PV is a chronic, autoimmune, supraepithelial blistering disease that affects mucosa and skin. The incidence of the disease is 0.1 to 0.5 per 100,000 people per year, with higher incidence in Ashkenazi Jews and Mediterranean individuals.[11] The

Table 1
Localized immunomodulatory agents for management of oral mucosal diseases

Therapies	Instructions
Steroidal Agents	

Gel/Cream/Ointment for Localized Lesions
    Fluocinonide gel 0.05%
    Clobetasol gel 0.05%
	• Use gauze to apply the gel to lesions 2–4 times daily, and keep the gauze in place for 5 min; do not eat for 30 min afterward
	• For gingival lesions, use occlusal trays to hold the gel against the oral mucosa

Oral Solutions for Diffuse/Difficult-to-reach Lesions
    Dexamethasone solution 0.5 mg/5 mL
    Prednisolone 3 mg/5 mL
	• Rinse with 5 mL for 3–5 min then expectorate, 2–4 times a day; do not drink or eat for 30 min afterward

Intralesional Injections for Localized Large Lesions Triamcinolone acetonide (10–40 mg/mL)	• Inject 0.1–0.2 mL/cm² just beneath the base of ulcers • Injections repeated weekly or every other week until complete healing
Nonsteroidal Agents	
Tacrolimus ointment 0.1%	• Use gauze to apply the ointment to lesions 2–4 times daily, and keep the gauze in place for 5 min; do not eat for 30 min afterward

disease is more common in women in their fifth to sixth decades of life.[3]

Pathobiology
The exact triggers are unknown. Circulating immunoglobulin (Ig) G autoantibodies are directed against specific cell-to-cell adhesion molecules in desmosomes, namely desmoglein-1 (Dsg-1) and desmoglein-3 (Dsg-3).[12] Dsg-3 is predominantly expressed in the mucosa, whereas Dsg-1 is mainly expressed in skin. Therefore, patients with mucosal disease have mainly anti–Dsg-3 antibodies that lead to suprabasal bullae formation and mucosal/skin acantholysis.[3,12]

Clinical manifestations
The oral mucosa is the first site of involvement in 50% of patients, preceding skin manifestations.[13,14] Oral lesions occur in almost 90% of patients during the course of disease.[13,15] Nasal, esophageal, laryngeal, anogenital, and conjunctival mucosa can be involved. Patients with oral involvement typically present with thin-walled bullae that rupture quickly into painful ulcers on the buccal and labial mucosa, palate, tongue, and gingiva (**Fig. 3**). DG can be present in less than one-third of patients.[3] Lesions may extend posteriorly to the larynx, oropharynx, and esophagus.[12] New blister formation caused by rubbing the normal mucosa, known as positive Nikolsky sign, is a common finding in PV but not pathognomonic.[12] Most patients ultimately present with skin lesions, manifested as flaccid bullae and erosions

on normal or erythematous skin of the trunk, groin, axillae, scalp, and face.[12] Progression of intraepithelial bullae formation can result in large areas of denuded skin and mucosa.[6] Secondary infection of the lesions is major complication of the disease caused by the loss of the epidermal/mucosal barrier and the immunocompromised state of the patients.[16]

Diagnosis
Clinical findings, routine histopathology, and immunofluorescence studies are necessary for accurate diagnosis.[17] Biopsy should be taken from the edge of the lesion and submitted for routine histopathology. A second perilesional biopsy from normal-appearing mucosal tissue is required for DIF.[12]

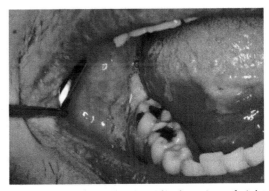

Fig. 3. Pemphigus vulgaris with ulceration of right buccal vestibule and the right ventrolateral tongue.

Histopathology

Histopathologic findings include suprabasilar clefting and acantholysis of keratinocytes. DIF shows intercellular deposition of IgG and C3 in a chicken-wire lattice pattern on the desmosomes between epithelial cells. Indirect immunofluorescence (IIF) and enzyme-linked immunosorbent assay (ELISA) are serologic tests usually performed to aid and/or confirm the diagnosis.[3] IIF uses an epithelial substrate to detect circulating autoantibodies against intracellular desmosomes, whereas ELISA is a sensitive test detecting the titer of specific circulating autoantibodies against Dsg1 and Dsg3 antigens in more than 90% of the cases.[11,13]

Management

Early diagnosis and treatment are necessary to control the severity of the disease.[13] Systemic corticosteroids remain the first-line treatment.[3] The treatment is supplemented with steroid-sparing agents, such as azathioprine, mycophenolate mofetil, and cyclophosphamide, to reduce the side effects of the steroids.[3,12] Rituximab, an anti-20 monoclonal antibody, has recently become the primary treatment of PV because of the low relapse rate and side effects.[12,18] The monoclonal antibody against B lymphocytes can effectively reduce the antibody production mediated by the disease.[12] Intravenous Ig (IVIG) can be used in combination with systemic steroids and/or immunosuppressive agents. Oral lesions are best managed in conjunction with systemic therapy or supplemented with high-potency topical corticosteroids alone (see **Table 1**).[12]

Mucous Membrane Pemphigoid

Epidemiology

MMP is a chronic, autoimmune, subepithelial blistering disease primarily affecting mucous membranes and infrequently the skin.[4] The estimated incidence of the diseases is between 1.3 and 2.0 per million per year and is more common in women between 60 and 80 years of age.[19,20]

Pathobiology

The cause of the disease remains unknown. Autoantibodies are directed against different hemidesmosomal antigens in the BMZ, including bullous pemphigoid antigen 1 (BPAg1 or BP230), bullous pemphigoid antigen 2 (BPAg2 or BP180), integrin subunits $\alpha6/\beta4$, laminin 311, laminin 332 (formerly known as laminin 5), and type VII collagen.[19] Around 50% to 70% of IgG and IgA autoantibodies were found against BP180 in patients with MMP.[3]

Clinical manifestations

Oral mucosa is often the initial site of involvement but this can be followed by involvement of the ocular mucosa.[20] The nasopharynx, esophagus, larynx, and the anogenital mucosa can be also affected. Oral lesions are present in approximately 85% of cases, characterized by fluid-filled bullae that rupture quickly leaving painful oral erosions and ulcers (**Fig. 4**). DG is the most common oral presentation of the disease.[3,21] Nikolsky sign can be positive in oral MMP. Skin lesions are uncommon, and present as recurrent vesicles and bullae on the face, neck, scalp, axilla, and extremities.[6,21] Extraoral lesions may heal with scarring, including ocular , which can lead to blindness.[19,20] However, oral mucosal lesions tend to heal without scarring.[3]

Diagnosis

Diagnosis is based on clinical findings, routine histopathology, and immunologic studies. Oral mucosal biopsies must be lesional/perilesional biopsy for routine hematoxylin-eosin and DIF studies.

Histopathology

Histopathology shows subepithelial clefting.[6] DIF shows linear deposition of IgG and C3, and sometimes IgA, at the BMZ. Serologic analysis by IIF and/or ELISA is used to detect autoantibodies against specific antigens in BMZ.[19,22]

Management

Topical corticosteroids are the mainstay treatment of oral MMP (see **Table 1**).[3] Systemic prednisone, steroid-sparing agents, and biologics are useful to control refractory cases and those with multifocal and/or systemic involvement. Dapsone and tetracycline are also among the therapeutic agents used for MMP.[3,19] Dapsone is a synthetic sulfone with antiinflammatory properties. The major side effect of dapsone is hemolytic anemia; thus,

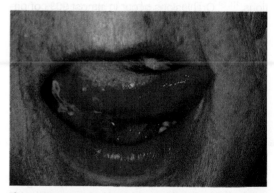

Fig. 4. Mucous membrane pemphigoid with multiple ulcerations of the right ventrolateral tongue.

patients should be screened for glucose-6-phosphate dehydrogenase (G6PD) deficiency before its initiation.[6,21] The tetracycline family is also known for its potent antiinflammatory effect. Because they have minimal side effects, they can be considered as safe alternatives to treat MMP.[6,20,21]

Linear Immunoglobulin A Disease

Epidemiology
Linear IgA disease is a rare, autoimmune, subepithelial blistering disease of skin and mucous membranes. The disease is most commonly seen in China, Africa, and Asia.[23,24] Women are more frequently affected than men in early childhood and in the sixth decade of life.[25]

Pathobiology
The cause is unknown. Different risk factors can trigger the immune response, such as drugs (vancomycin), infections, trauma, autoimmune diseases, and malignancies. IgA autoantibodies target antigens in hemidesmosomes, mainly BP180/collagen XVII.[25,26]

Clinical manifestations
Oral and ocular mucosa are the most commonly affected sites.[25] Oral findings include vesiculobullous eruptions that rupture quickly into painful ulcers and erosions. White reticulations, erythema, and DG are common.[23,26] Oral lesions do not scar; however, ocular scarring may lead to blindness.[26] Children can present with pruritic vesicles and bullae on an erythematous or normal skin mostly on the lower abdomen, perineal area, and inner thighs, whereas the same lesions can be seen on the trunk in adults.[24,27]

Diagnosis
Diagnosis is based on routine histopathology and immunofluorescence studies.

Histopathology
Histopathologic examination shows subepithelial clefting. DIF shows linear deposition of IgA on the BMZ, with IgG and C3 deposition in some cases. IIF is usually negative for circulating IgA autoantibodies against BMZ.[26]

Management
Dapsone is considered the first line of treatment.[25] Screening for glucose-6-phosphate dehydrogenase (G6PD) deficiency via blood test should be completed before initiation of dapsone therapy to avoid hemolytic anemia. Other medications, such as systemic corticosteroid, sulfapyridine, cyclophosphamide, mycophenolate mofetil, tetracycline, and colchicine, can be effective to control

disease.[25] Oral lesions are best managed with topical corticosteroids (see **Table 1**).

Epidermolysis Bullosa

Epidemiology
Epidermolysis bullosa (EB) is a group of inherited, chronic, blistering diseases characterized by fragility of skin and mucous membranes, resulting in blister formation after minor trauma or irritation. Lesions occurs at birth or early childhood with no sex predilection. The disease is rare, with an incidence of approximately 1 in 50,000 live births.[28] A disorder termed EB acquisita is an autoimmune condition that clinically resembles the inherited EB, affecting middle-aged and older adults rather than children[29,30]

Pathobiology
Mutations of specific proteins in skin and mucous membrane, including keratin 5 and 14, laminin332, collagen type VII and XVII, and α6 β4 integrin, have been implicated in the development of the disease.[28]

Clinical manifestations
Patients present with oral blisters that heal with scar, resulting in microstomia and ankyloglossia. Reduction of vestibular depth and atrophy of jaw bones have been reported.[31] Dental abnormalities, such as enamel hypoplasia, anodontia, periodontitis, and dental caries, can be associated with the disease. Cutaneous vesiculobullous lesions are also common and tend to heal with scarring.

Diagnosis
Diagnosis is based on clinical presentation and histopathologic findings.

Histopathology
Histopathologic examination shows blister formation at different levels of the dermal-epidermal junction.[29]

Management
There is no definitive treatment of the disease. Patients with EB have a higher risk of developing caries. Oral hygiene instruction, brushing with soft toothbrushes, and fluoride application are recommended to control dental caries.[32] A dietary consultation is important to prevent caries and should be initiated at an early age.[33]

Lupus Erythematosus

Epidemiology
Lupus erythematosus (LE) is a group of chronic, autoimmune diseases with a wide range of relapsing and remitting clinical abnormalities affecting different organs and tissues.[34] Two forms of the

disease are associated with oral lesions: systemic LE (SLE), and cutaneous or discoid LE (DLE).[35] SLE is reported more frequently in African American women of childbearing age, with the true incidence being unknown.[36,37]

Pathobiology

The cause of the disease is still unclear. Environmental, genetic, and hormonal abnormalities may be associated with pathogenesis.[37] Ultraviolet light is a known trigger for DLE.[38] Autoantibodies produced against DNA and other nuclear antigens are characteristic. In SLE, deposition of immune complexes in tissues and organs is associated with organ failure, whereas, in DLE, deposition of immune complexes in the dermal-epidermal junction leads to skin inflammation[38,39] In addition, 80% of the patients present with autoantibodies against endothelial cells, resulting in vasculitis.[40]

Clinical manifestations

DLE is a localized disease characterized by discoid, erythematous plaques with hyperkeratosis on the skin or/and mucosa, whereas SLE can involve any organ of the body, with the patients having a wide range of symptoms from mild fever, fatigue, arthralgia/arthritis, and butterfly rash to severe debilitating disease with cardiac, renal, and neurologic complications.[35,39,41] Oral lesions can present in both types of the disease. Approximately 25% of patients with DLE present with oral lesions, whereas up to 40% of patients with SLE have oral involvement.[36] Oral findings include unilateral distribution of lichenoid lesions on the tongue, hard palate, or the vermilion borders of the lips.[37,39]

Diagnosis

Diagnosis is based on the clinical findings, together with serology and biopsy. The European League Against Rheumatism (EULAR) and the American College of Rheumatology (ACR) have developed the classification criteria for SLE. Positive antinuclear antibodies, anti–double-stranded DNA, and anti-Smith antibodies are the serologic markers to establish the diagnosis.[5,42]

Histopathology

Histopathologic findings are mainly of lichenoid mucositis similar to OLP.[43] However, deep perivascular inflammation presents more frequently in LE.[36] DIF shows IgG, IgM, and IgA, with or without C3 deposition in a granular pattern at the BMZ. This finding is known as positive lupus band.[29]

Management

Management is determined according to the severity and extent of the disease.[39] Patients can be managed by using a combination of nonsteroidal antiinflammatory drugs, antimalarials (hydroxychloroquine), systemic corticosteroids (prednisone), and immunosuppressive drugs such as azathioprine, mycophenolate mofetil, and methotrexate. Recently, biologic agents such as belimumab have been approved for SLE.[34] Topical corticosteroids in conjunction with intralesional steroid injections or topical tacrolimus are effective for oral lesions (see **Table 1**).[39]

Behcet Disease

Epidemiology

Behcet disease (BD) is a rare, autoimmune, multisystemic disease affecting the blood vessels of almost all organs. The disease occurs worldwide, with the highest prevalence in Turkey and the Middle East.[44] Men are more frequently affected than women, with peak of incidence between second and fourth decades of life.[44]

Pathobiology

The cause of the disease remains unknown. Genetics is an important risk factor in the pathogenesis of the disease, with the *HLA-B51* genetic marker being associated with 15% to 80% of patients; however, the exact role of *HLA-B51* in the pathogenesis is unknown.[44,45]

Clinical manifestations

The presence of oral aphthous ulcers and 2 of the following are required for the diagnosis of BD: recurrent genital ulcers, ocular inflammation, skin lesions, and positive pathergy test.[46,47] Oral recurrent aphthous stomatitis (RAS) is the most common finding, seen in 97% to 100% of the patients, and is characterized by well-defined small ulcers surrounded by erythematous halo (**Fig. 5**).[44,48] Lesions present as single or multiple ulcers on nonkeratinized mucosa, including buccal/labial mucosa and ventral/lateral tongue.[45,48] Approximately 80% of patients present with skin lesions such as erythema nodosum–like lesions and erythema multiforme–like rashes.[47] Pathergy test is usually positive, with positivity rates varying according to geographic areas.[47] The test describes hyperactivity reaction characterized by pustulopapular eruptions in the skin after 24 to 48 hours of intracutaneous needle injection.[47]

Diagnosis

Patients are diagnosed based on clinical manifestations and by excluding other conditions associated with RAS.[49] Because of the strong association between BD and human leukocyte

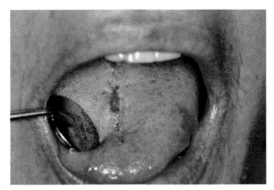

Fig. 5. Aphthous ulcers on the left dorsum tongue in patient with Behçet disease.

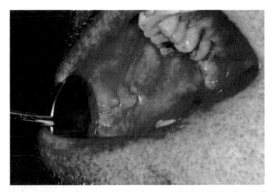

Fig. 6. Ulceration and erythema of the right buccal mucosa in a patient with chronic graft-versus-host disease.

antigen (HLA) B51 positivity, testing for HLA-B51 can be considered.[50]

Histopathology
Histopathologic features are not specific, showing ulcerative lesions covered by fibrin.[47]

Management
Topical corticosteroids and intralesional steroids are useful to treat painful oral ulcers (see **Table 1**).[45] Various systemic drugs can be used, such as prednisone, colchicine, thalidomide, pentoxifylline, azathioprine, apremilast, and anti–tumor necrosis factor inhibitors.[29]

Chronic Graft-Versus-Host Disease

Epidemiology
Chronic graft-versus-host disease (cGVHD) is a multisystemic, immune-mediated complication occurring in 30% to 70% of patients undergoing allogenic hematopoietic stem cell transplant.[51] The condition frequently involves the liver, skin, eyes, lungs, and oral cavity.[51,52] It may occur after acute graft-versus-host disease; however, around 30% of cases occur without an acute presentation.[53]

Pathobiology
Donor T cells react against host antigens, resulting in immune response and deposition of immune complexes in host tissue causing inflammation and fibrosis.[51] Different risk factors, such as HLA incompatibility, advanced age, gender mismatching, and the use of peripheral blood, are associated with an increased risk of developing cGVHD.[54]

Clinical manifestations
Oral mucosa is affected in approximately 80% of the patients.[52] Oral mucosal lesions of cGVHD are characterized by erythema, ulcers, hyperkeratotic plaques, and lichenoid lesions, particularly involving the tongue and buccal mucosa (**Fig. 6**).[55,56] Salivary glands are commonly affected, resulting in xerostomia and subsequent

caries and fungal infection. Superficial mucoceles can occur on the palatal mucosa and other sites of minor salivary glands (**Fig. 7**). Sclerotic skin or mucosal fibrosis may lead to limited mouth opening.[57] Patients with cGVHD are at increased risk of developing secondary oral squamous cell carcinoma.[58] Skin manifestations range from lichenoid lesions to skin sclerosis, with common features including depigmentation, poikiloderma, erythema, maculopapular rash, and pruritus.[51,59]

Diagnosis
Diagnosis is based on history and clinical findings and may be aided by histologic examination. Oral swabs for viral testing may be necessary to differentiate between oral cGVHD and recrudescent herpes simplex virus.[56]

Histopathology
Histopathologic features resemble those of OLP. In advanced cases, collagen deposition can be seen, similar to systemic sclerosis. A specimen of minor salivary glands shows a periductal lymphocytic infiltration.[60]

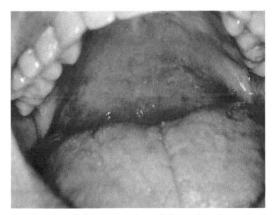

Fig. 7. Superficial mucoceles of the palate in patient with chronic graft-versus-host disease.

Management

Management is based on the severity and extent of the disease. Systemic corticosteroid therapy is the first line of treatment of systemic disease, often in combination with immunomodulatory agents (tacrolimus, cyclosporine, mycophenolate mofetil, and azathioprine) to mitigate the side effects of long-term use of corticosteriods.[54] In severe cases, increased dosage or a new systemic immunosuppressive is required.[56] Biologics such as monoclonal antibodies (rituximab) and tyrosine kinase inhibitors (imatinib, ibrutinib, ruxolitinib) can be also used. Ibrutinib is the first US Food and Drug Administration (FDA)–approved treatment of cGVHD.[52] Extracorporeal photopheresis may be effective in refractory cases.[52] Lesions limited to the oral cavity can be sufficiently managed with topical and localized immunomodulatory therapy (see **Table 1**). Frequent hydration, salivary substitutes, and sialagogues are used to alleviate xerostomia.[60] Patients at risk to develop carious lesions require prescription fluoride, to maintain good oral hygiene, and to avoid cariogenic foods and drinks.[52,56] In addition, patients with cGVHD are susceptible to develop oral squamous cell carcinoma, and therefore long-term follow-up and biopsy are required for any suspicions lesions.[52,56]

CHRONIC REACTIVE LESIONS
Frictional Keratosis

Epidemiology

Oral white lesions are frequently encountered in daily dental practice. These lesions are usually associated with mechanical irritation such as brushing, biting, or rubbing of teeth against oral mucosa.[24]

Clinical manifestations

Chronic irritation to oral mucosa produces poorly defined, unilateral or bilateral, white plaques or papules. Oral frictional keratosis can present on buccal mucosa, labial mucosa, or lateral tongue. In addition, a masticatory force or trauma from ill-fitting dentures may cause ill-defined white plaques or papules on the retromolar area and edentulous alveolar ridge, known as benign alveolar ridge keratosis (**Fig. 8**).[61,62]

Diagnosis

Diagnosis is based on clinical presentation. Biopsy and histopathologic examination may be necessary in atypical cases.

Histopathology

Histopathologic findings include hyperkeratosis, acanthosis, ragged epithelial surface with keratin projections, and bacterial colonies.[63]

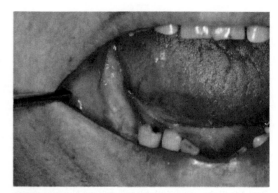

Fig. 8. Benign alveolar ridge keratosis.

Management

No treatment is required. Lesions are usually reversible in 2 weeks after cessation of parafunctional habit or elimination of source of trauma. If lesions still persist and diagnosis is uncertain, biopsy may be indicated.[29,62]

Smokeless Tobacco Keratosis

Epidemiology

Smokeless tobacco keratosis (known as snuff dipper's lesion, tobacco pouch keratosis, and spit tobacco keratosis) is a reactive lesion at the site where the smokeless tobacco has been placed. Lesions present in 15% of individuals using chewing tobacco, and in 60% of snuff tobacco users.[29,64] Risk of malignant transformation to squamous cell carcinoma is less than 3%.[65]

Clinical manifestations

Wrinkled, white to gray plaques are mostly observed in the mandibular labial and buccal mucosa (**Fig. 9**). Depending on quantity and frequency

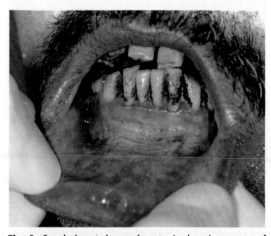

Fig. 9. Smokeless tobacco keratosis showing areas of keratosis and wrinkling of anterior mandibular vestibule. (*Courtesy of* Binmadi N and Almazrooa S, Oral and maxillofacial Pathology, King Abdulaziz University Faculty of Dentistry, Jeddah, Saudi Arabia.)

of smokeless tobacco exposure, white areas become thickened, leathery, and nodular.[29,66]

Diagnosis

Diagnosis is based on clinical presentation and histopathologic findings.

Histopathology

Histopathologic features include hyperkeratosis and acanthosis with or without vacuolization of the mucosal epithelium. Parakeratin chevrons can be seen in the keratin surface. Inflammation and deposition of amorphous eosinophilic material is noted in connective tissue.[29]

Management

Lesions are reversible in weeks after discontinuation of the habit. Excisional biopsy is necessary to rule out malignancy if the lesions persist.

Nicotine Stomatitis

Epidemiology

Nicotine stomatitis, or smoker's palate, presents as diffuse palatal changes associated with pipe or cigar smoking and develops in response to the heat generated from the tobacco smoke. A reverse smoker's palate is a more severe form of nicotine stomatitis seen more in southern Asia and South American countries and is highly associated with malignant transformation.[67]

Clinical manifestations

Diffuse, thickened, gray to white plaques with a fissured surface present on the palatal mucosa (**Fig. 10**). Numerous papules with central red dots can be observed, representing inflamed orifices of minor salivary glands ducts.[5]

Diagnosis

Diagnosis is based on clinical presentation and histopathologic findings.

Histopathology

Histopathologic features include hyperkeratosis, acanthosis, and squamous metaplasia of the minor salivary glands' duct orifices.[29]

Management

Smoker's palate is reversible with smoking cessation. Lesions that persist require biopsy.

Irritation Fibroma

Epidemiology

Irritation fibroma is the most common tumorlike lesion of the oral cavity.[68] It represents a benign hyperplasia of fibrous connective tissue as a result of trauma or irritation to oral mucosa. Other chronic exophytic lesions can be encountered in the oral cavity, such as peripheral ossifying fibroma, pyogenic granuloma, peripheral giant cell granuloma, and traumatic neuroma (**Fig. 11**, **Table 2**).[29,68,69]

Clinical manifestations

Clinically, fibromas usually manifest asymptomatic, firm, sessile, pale pink nodules, similar to the surrounding oral mucosa. The surface is smooth, but it can be ulcerated or hyperkeratotic because of trauma. Common sites include the buccal mucosa, lower labial mucosa, and lateral tongue, with lesions ranging from a few millimeters to 1.5 cm in diameter.[68,70]

Diagnosis

Diagnosis is based on clinical presentation and histopathologic features.

Histopathology

Histopathologic examination shows a nodular mass of dense fibrous connective tissue with scattered chronic inflammatory cells.[29]

Management

Bothersome irritation fibromas can be managed with conservative surgical excision; however,

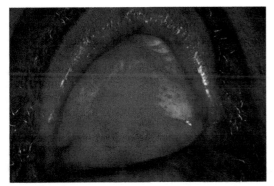

Fig. 10. Nicotine stomatitis showing a diffuse erythematous area with small papules representing inflamed orifices of minor salivary glands ducts.

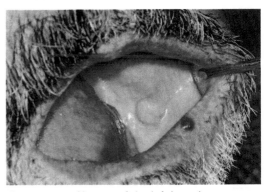

Fig. 11. Large fibroma of the left buccal mucosa.

Table 2
Oral exophytic reactive lesions

Reactive Lesions	Epidemiology	Clinical Manifestations	Histopathology	Management
Epulis fissuratum	• No sex predilection • Middle-aged and older adults	• Asymptomatic • Firm, 1 or more hyperplastic folds • Surface is smooth, can be erythematous or ulcerated • In the maxillary alveolar vestibule	Mass of fibrovascular connective tissue hyperplasia	Surgical excision Refabrication or relining of ill-fitting denture
Irritation fibroma	• F>M • Fourth to sixth decades	• Asymptomatic • Firm, sessile nodules • Surface is smooth, can be ulcerated or hyperkeratotic • Pale pink • On buccal, lower labial mucosa and lateral tongue • Size varies from millimeters to 1–2 cm	Mass of fibrous connective tissue	Surgical excision
Peripheral ossifying fibroma	• F>M • Second decade	• Asymptomatic • Firm, pedunculated or sessile nodules • Surface is smooth, often ulcerated • On the gingiva, mainly arises from the interdental papilla • Red to pink • Size is <2 cm	Mass of fibrous connective tissue with scattered mineralization	Surgical excision
Pyogenic granuloma (lobular capillary hemangioma)	• F>M • Children and young adults	• Asymptomatic • Soft to firm, pedunculated or sessile nodules • Surface is smooth or lobulated, often ulcerated and bleeds • On gingiva • Red or yellow • Size varies from millimeters to several centimeters	Lobulated mass of vascular proliferation	Surgical excision
Peripheral giant cell granuloma	• F>M • Fourth to sixth decades	• Asymptomatic • Firm, smooth, pedunculated or sessile nodules • On gingiva/edentulous alveolar mucosa • Dark red to bluish purple • Size is <2 cm, can be larger	Mass of multinucleated cells in cellular and vascular stroma	Surgical excision

(continued on next page)

Table 2
(continued)

Reactive Lesions	Epidemiology	Clinical Manifestations	Histopathology	Management
Traumatic neuroma	• F>M • Middle aged	• Painful • Smooth, nodular mass • In mental foramen area, lower lip and tongue	Mass of haphazardly arranged nerve bundles, within a collagenous and fibroblastic stroma	Surgical excision

Abbreviations: F, female; M, male.

lesions do not require removal. Fibromas have a low recurrence rate.[68]

GENETIC LESIONS
White Sponge Nevus

Epidemiology
White sponge nevus (WSN) is also known as Cannon disease, an autosomal dominant disorder characterized by abnormal keratinization of mucous membranes, primarily affecting the oral mucosa.[46] It is a rare disease, with an estimated incidence of 1 in 200,000.[71] Lesions usually present at birth or during early childhood with no sex predilection.[29]

Pathobiology
Mutations of keratin 4 and/or keratin 13 genes in the spinous cell layer have been attributed to the development of WSN.[71]

Clinical manifestations
Oral lesions are characterized by asymptomatic, symmetric, white plaques with corrugated or fissured surface (**Fig. 12**). Bilateral buccal mucosa is the most commonly affected site, followed by labial mucosa, soft palate, ventral tongue, and floor of the mouth.[69]

Diagnosis
Diagnosis is based on clinical presentation and histopathologic findings.

Histopathology
Histopathologic examination shows hyperkeratosis with vacuolization of epithelial cells. Aggregation of keratin in the form of perinuclear eosinophilic condensation is a characteristic feature of the disease.[29]

Management
No treatment is necessary.

INFECTIOUS CHRONIC ORAL LESIONS
Oral Candidiasis

Epidemiology and pathobiology
Oral candidiasis is the most common oral fungal infection and is typically caused by *Candida albicans*.[29] *Candida* is a component of normal oral flora in 60% of healthy individuals.[1] Disturbance of the oral flora by factors such as reduced salivary flow, use of steroid inhalers or antibiotics, use of dentures, smoking, and immunosuppression has been shown to increase risk of oral candidiasis.[72]

Clinical manifestations
The disease has a wide variety of clinical presentations. Chronic conditions are rarely observed and

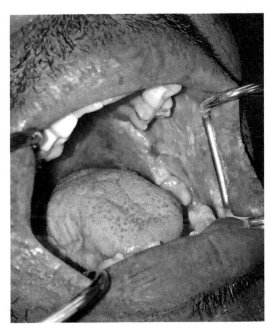

Fig. 12. White sponge nevus of the left buccal mucosa. (*Courtesy of* Muller S., MD Atlanta Oral Pathology, Emory University School of Medicine, Decatur, GA.)

usually occur in the context of immunosuppression and salivary gland dysfunction. The most common 3 variants of oral candidiasis are pseudomembranous candidiasis, erythematous candidiasis, and chronic hyperplastic candidiasis. Pseudomembranous candidiasis, referred to as thrush, is the most common clinical presentation of oral candidiasis. Chronic lesions characterized by white or yellow creamy plaques (so-called cottage-cheese appearance) occur at any site in the oral cavity. These lesions can be wiped off, leaving an erythematous surface with minimal bleeding.[5,73] In chronic erythematous candidiasis, patients present with erythematous macules/papules on dorsal tongue and hard palate. Chronic lesions of pseudomembranous or erythematous candidiasis are asymptomatic. However, they are occasionally associated with a burning sensation and altered taste.[73] Chronic hyperplastic candidiasis is characterized by a well-demarcated, white plaque, most often on anterior buccal mucosa.[73] Lesions cannot be scraped off and are clinically indistinguishable from leukoplakia.[1]

Diagnosis

Diagnosis is based on clinical findings. Cytologic smear can help confirm the diagnosis. Fungal culture and sensitivity test can be performed if lesions are not responsive to empiric antifungal therapy. Biopsy is required for diagnosis of chronic hyperplastic candidiasis to rule out dysplasia.[5]

Histopathology

Histopathologic findings include *Candida* hyphae on the epithelial surface.[29]

Management

Management of oral candidiasis includes both topical and systemic strategies (**Table 3**). Patients who wear dentures should be advised to remove them at bedtime and soak in commercially available denture cleansers or in chlorohexidine. Predisposing factors should be identified and managed properly.[5,74] Long-term prophylaxis may be necessary in some cases with recurrent infections.

ORAL LESIONS ASSOCIATED WITH HUMAN PAPILLOMA VIRUS
Epidemiology and Pathobiology

Human papilloma virus (HPV) is a group of double-stranded DNA viruses that infect epithelium and induce the formation of a variety of benign and malignant epithelial lesions of the upper digestive and anogenital mucosa. More than 220 HPV subtypes have been identified, of which more than 30 types are known to infect the oral mucosa.[29,75] HPV 16 and 18 have been associated with oropharyngeal squamous cell carcinoma and cervical cancer.[75]

Clinical Variants

Benign oral lesions associated with HPV include squamous papilloma, verruca vulgaris, and condyloma acuminatum (**Table 4**). These lesions can generally be diagnosed clinically and do not require excision unless sufficiently bothersome (**Fig. 13**).[5,29,76]

Prevention

Three FDA-approved vaccinations are available to prevent HPV infection (Cervarix, Gardasil-4, Gardasil-9).[75] The use of Gardasil-4 is discontinued in the United States. Cervarix is recommended for female patients between 9 and 25 years of age and protects against high oncogenic HPV types (16 and 18), whereas Gardasil-9 is approved for both male and female patients between 9 and 26 years old, and protects against HPV 16, 18, 6, and 11 in addition to HPV 31, 33, 45, 52, 58.[75]

Table 3
Antifungal therapy for oral candidiasis

Antifungal	Instructions
Topical	
Clotrimazole troche 10 mg	Dissolve the troche in the mouth 4–5 times a day, for 7–14 d
Nystatin suspension 100,000 U/mL	Swish 5 mL for 2–3 min and then spit 4 times daily, for 7–14 d
For angular cheilitis: nystatin 100,000 U/mL combined with triamcinolone acetonide 1% cream	Apply to the corners of the mouth twice daily, until the lesion resolves
Systemic	
Fluconazole 100 mg	Take 1 tablet daily, for 1–2 wk

Table 4
Oral lesions associated with human papilloma virus

Oral Lesions	Epidemiology	Clinical Manifestations	Histopathology	Management

Squamous papilloma	• M>F
	• 30–50 y
	• Associated with HPV 6, 11
		• Asymptomatic
		• Pedunculated nodule, with fingerlike (papillary) projections
		• Pink or white
		• On palate or tongue
		• The size is <0.5 cm but can be larger
			Epithelial proliferation arranged in fingerlike projections with fibrovascular connective tissue core	• Complete surgical excision
				• Other treatment modalities such as:
				  ○ Electrocautery
				  ○ Cryosurgery
				  ○ Intralesional interferon

Verruca vulgaris (common warts)	• No sex predilection • 12–16 y • Associated with HPV 2	• Asymptomatic • Sessile, or pedunculated nodules with papillary projections • White, pink, or yellow • On vermilion border, labial mucosa, or anterior tongue • The size is <5 mm	Epithelial proliferation arranged in fingerlike pointed projections with connective tissue core and elongated rete ridges toward the center	
Condyloma acuminatum (venereal warts)	• No sex predilection • Adolescence and young adults • Associated with HPV 6, 11	• Asymptomatic • Sessile nodule with papillary projections • Pink • On labial mucosa, lingual frenum, and soft palate • Size reaches 1.5–3 cm	Proliferation of acanthotic epithelium arranged in blunt, broad, fingerlike projections with thin connective tissue core	

Gardasil-9 is used to prevent oral HPV infections as well as oropharyngeal cancers. Therefore, early HPV vaccination before the onset of sexual activity is recommended for both female and male patients to decrease the risk of HPV infection.[75,77] Recently, the FDA approved the use of Gardasil-9 HPV vaccine in women and men aged 27 through 45 years in order to reduce the occurrence of new HPV infections in adults.[78]

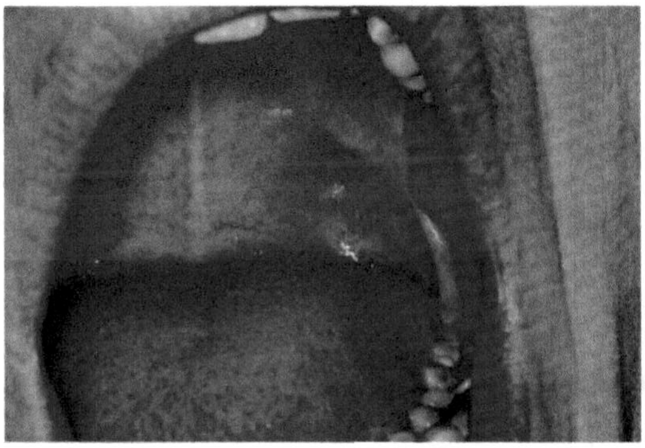

SUMMARY

There is a wide clinical spectrum of chronic oral mucosal lesions that may be encountered in the dermatology clinic. Appropriate management depends on an accurate diagnosis. Patients with such conditions may benefit from interdisciplinary care between dermatology and oral medicine to ensure optimal outcomes.

DISCLOSURE

This article represents an original writing that is not being considered for publication elsewhere. All authors have read and approved the article. The authors report no conflicts of interest related to the content of this article.

Fig. 13. Squamous papilloma on the soft palate.

REFERENCES

1. Stoopler E, Sollecito TP. Oral mucosal diseases: evaluation and management. Med Clin North Am 2014;98(6):1323–52.
2. Crincoli V, Di Bisceglie MB, Scivetti M, et al. Oral lichen planus: update on etiopathogenesis, diagnosis and treatment. Immunopharmacol Immunotoxicol 2011;33(1):11–20.
3. Kuten-Shorrer M, Menon RS, Lerman MA. Mucocutaneous Diseases. Dent Clin North Am 2020;64(1):139–62.
4. Li D, Li J, Li C, et al. The Association of Thyroid Disease and Oral Lichen Planus: A Literature Review and Meta-analysis. Front Endocrinol (Lausanne) 2017;8:310.
5. Bruch JM, Treister NS. Clinical oral medicine and pathology. 2nd edition. New York: Springer; 2017.
6. Stoopler ET, Sollecito TP, DeRossi SS. Desquamative gingivitis: Early presenting symptom of mucocutaneous disease. Quintessence Int 2003;34(8):582–6.
7. Au J, Patel D, Campbell JH. Oral lichen planus. Oral Maxillofac Surg Clin 2013;25(1):93–100.
8. Cheng YS, Gould A, Kurago Z, et al. Diagnosis of oral lichen planus: a position paper of the American Academy of Oral and Maxillofacial Pathology. Oral Surg Oral Med Oral Pathol Oral Radiol 2016;122(3):332–54.
9. Gorouhi F, Davari P, Fazel N. Cutaneous and mucosal lichen planus: a comprehensive review of clinical subtypes, risk factors, diagnosis, and prognosis. ScientificWorldJournal 2014;2014:742826.
10. De Rossi SS, Ciarrocca K. Oral lichen planus and lichenoid mucositis. Dent Clin North Am 2014;58(2):299–313.
11. McMillan R, Taylor J, Shephard M, et al. World workshop on oral medicine VI: a systematic review of the treatment of mucocutaneous pemphigus vulgaris. Oral Surg Oral Med Oral Pathol Oral Radiol 2015;120(2):132–42.
12. Santoro FA, Stoopler ET, Werth VP. Pemphigus. Dent Clin North Am 2013;5(4):597–610.
13. Porro AM, Seque CA, Ferreira MCC, et al. Pemphigus vulgaris. An Bras Dermatol 2019;94(3):264–78.
14. Robinson JC, Lozada-Nur F, Frieden I. Oral pemphigus vulgaris: a review of the literature and a report on the management of 12 cases. Oral Surg Oral Med Oral Pathol Oral Radiol Endod 1997;84(4):349–55.
15. Kumar SJ, Nehru Anand SP, Gunasekaran N, et al. Oral pemphigus vulgaris: A case report with direct immunofluorescence study. J Oral Maxillofac Pathol 2016;20(3):549.
16. Esmaili N, Mortazavi H, Noormohammadpour P, et al. Pemphigus vulgaris and infections: a retrospective study on 155 patients. Autoimmun Dis 2013;2013:834295.
17. Scully C, Challacombe SJ. Pemphigus vulgaris: update on etiopathogenesis, oral manifestations, and management. Rev Oral Biol Med 2002;13(5):397–408.
18. Fortuna G, Calabria E, Ruoppo E, et al. The use of rituximab as an adjuvant in the treatment of oral pemphigus vulgaris. J Oral Pathol Med 2020;49:91–5.
19. Taylor J, McMillan R, Shephard M, et al. World workshop on oral medicine VI: a systematic review of the treatment of mucous membrane pemphigoid. Oral Surg Oral Med Oral Pathol Oral Radiol 2015;120(2):161–71.
20. Xu HH, Werth VP, Parisi E, et al. Mucous membrane pemphigoid. Dent Clin North Am 2013;57(4):611–30.
21. Scully C, Lo Muzio L. Oral mucosal diseases: Mucous membrane pemphigoid. Br J Oral Maxillofac Surg 2008;46(5):358–66.
22. Kamaguchi M, Iwata H. The diagnosis and blistering mechanisms of mucous membrane pemphigoid. Front Immunol 2019;10:34.
23. Lewis MA, Yaqoob NA, Emanuel C, et al. Successful treatment of oral linear IgA disease using mycophenolate. Oral Surg Oral Med Oral Pathol Oral Radiol Endod 2007;103(4):483–6.
24. Venning VA. Linear IgA disease: clinical presentation, diagnosis, and pathogenesis. Immunol Allergy Clin N Am 2012;32(2):245–53.
25. Chaudhari S, Mobini N. Linear IgA bullous dermatosis a rare clinicopathologic entity with an unusual presentation. J Clin Aesthet Dermatol 2015;8(10):43–6.
26. Joseph TI, Sathyan P, Goma Kumar KU. Linear IgA dermatosis adult variant with oral manifestation: A rare case report. J Oral Maxillofac Pathol 2015;19(1):83–7.
27. Leuci S, Ruoppo E, Adamo D, et al. Oral autoimmune vesicobullous diseases: classification, clinical presentations, molecular mechanisms, diagnostic algorithms, and management. Periodontol 2000 2019;80(1):7–11.
28. Maldonado-Colin G, Hernández-Zepeda C, Duran-McKinster C, et al. Inherited epidermolysis bullosa: a multisystem disease of skin and mucosae. Indian J Paediatr Dermatol 2017;18:267–73.
29. Neville B, Douglas DD, Allen CM, et al. Oral and maxillofacial pathology. 4th edition. St Louis (MO): Elsevier; 2016.
30. Ludwig RJ. Clinical presentation, pathogenesis, diagnosis, and treatment of epidermolysis bullosa Acquisita. ISRN Dermatol 2013;2013:812029.
31. Dag C, Bezgin T, Özalp N. Dental management of patients with epidermolysis bullosa. Oral Health Dent Manag 2014;13(3):623–7.

32. Esfahanizade K, Mahdavi AR, Ansari G, et al. Epidermolysis bullosa, dental and anesthetic management: a case report. J Dent (Shiraz) 2014;15(3):147–52.

33. Krämer SM, Serrano MC, Zillmann G, et al. Oral health care for patients with epidermolysis bullosa - best clinical practice guidelines. Int J Paediatr Dent 2012;22(Suppl. 1):1–35.

34. Bernknopf A, Rak K, Bailey T. A review of systemic lupus erythematosus and current treatment options. Formulary 2011;46:178–94.

35. Bugueno JM, Alawi F, Stoopler ER. Asymptomatic oral mucosal lesions. J Am Dent Assoc 2013; 144(9):1010–3.

36. Jorizzo JL, Salisbury PL, Rogers RS 3rd, et al. Oral lesions in systemic lupus erythematosus. Do ulcerative lesions represent a necrotizing vasculitis? J Am Acad Dermatol 1992;27(3):389–94.

37. Louis PJ, Fernandes R. Review of systemic lupus erythematosus. Oral Surg Oral Med Oral Pathol Oral Radiol Endod 2001;91(5):512–6.

38. Stannard JN, Kahlenberg JM. Cutaneous lupus erythematosus: updates on pathogenesis and associations with systemic lupus. Curr Opin Rheumatol 2017;28(5):453–9.

39. Fortuna G, Brennan MT. Systemic lupus erythematosus epidemiology, pathophysiology, manifestations, and management. Dent Clin North Am 2013;57(4):631–55.

40. Cieślik P, Hrycek A, Kłuciński P. Vasculopathy and vasculitis in systemic lupus erythematosus. Pol Arch Med Wewn 2008;118(1–2):57–63.

41. Kuhn A, Bonsmann G, Anders HJ, et al. The diagnosis and treatment of systemic lupus erythematosus. Dtsch Arztebl Int 2015;112(25):423–32.

42. Aringer M, Costenbader K, Daikh D, et al. 2019 European League Against Rheumatism/American College of Rheumatology classification criteria for systemic lupus erythematosus. Arthritis Rheumatol 2019;71(9):1400–12.

43. Lourenxco SV, de Carvalho FR, Boggio P, et al. Lupus erythematosus: Clinical and histopathological study of oral manifestations and immunohistochemical profile of the inflammatory infiltrate. J Cutan Pathol 2007;34(7):558–64.

44. Nair JR, Moots RJ. Behçet's disease. Clin Med 2017; 17(1):71–7.

45. Stoopler ET, Mirfarsi S, Alawi F, et al. Recalcitrant gingival lesions in a patient previously diagnosed with Behçet's disease. Compend Contin Educ Dent 2019;40(1):46–8.

46. Ideguchi H, Suda A, Takeno M, et al. Behcet disease: evolution of clinical manifestations. Medicine (Baltimore) 2011;90(2):125–32.

47. Kokturk A. Clinical and pathological manifestations with differential diagnosis in Behcet's disease. Patholog Res Int 2012;2012:690390.

48. Rokutanda R, Kishimoto M, Okada M. Update on the diagnosis and management of Behcet's disease. Open Access Rheumatol 2015;7:1–8.

49. International Team for the Revision of the International Criteria for Behçet's Disease (ITR-ICBD). The International Criteria for Behçet's Disease (ICBD): a collaborative study of 27 countries on the sensitivity and specificity of the new criteria. J Eur Acad Dermatol Venereol 2014;28(3):338–47.

50. Menthon MD, Lavalley MP, Maldini C, et al. HLA–B51/B5 and the risk of Behçet's disease: a systematic review and meta-analysis of case–control genetic association studies. Arthritis Rheum 2009; 61(10):1287–96.

51. Jagasia MH, Greinix HT, Arora M, et al. National Institutes of Health consensus development project on criteria for clinical trials in chronic graft-versus-host disease: I. the 2014 diagnosis and staging working group report. Biol Blood Marrow Transplant 2015;21(3):389–401.e1.

52. Mawardi H, Hashmi SK, Elad S, et al. Chronic graft-versus-host disease: Current management paradigm and future perspectives. Oral Dis 2019;25:931–48.

53. Lee SJ. Classification systems for chronic graft-versus-host disease. Blood 2017;129(1):30–7.

54. Kuten-Shorrer M, Woo SB, Treister NS. Oral graft-versus-host disease. Dent Clin North Am 2014; 75(2):351–68.

55. Castellarin P, Stevenson K, Biasotto M, et al. Extensive dental caries in patients with oral chronic graft-versus-host disease. Biol Blood Marrow Transplant 2012;18(10):1573–9.

56. Treister N, Duncan C, Cutler C, et al. How we treat oral chronic graft-versus-host disease. Blood 2012; 120(17):3407–18.

57. Elad S, Jensen SB, Raber-Durlacher JE, et al. Clinical approach in the management of oral chronic graft-versus-host disease (cGVHD) in a series of specialized medical centers. Support Care Cancer 2015;23(6):1615–22.

58. Majhail NS. Secondary cancers following allogeneic haematopoietic cell trans-plantation in adults. Br J Haematol 2011;154(3):301–10.

59. Ratanatharathorn V, Ayash L, Lazarus HM, et al. Chronic graft-versus-host disease: clinical manifestation and therapy. Bone Marrow Transplant 2001;28:121–9.

60. Hull K, Kerridge I, Avery S, et al. Oral chronic graft-versus-host disease in Australia: clinical features and challenges in management. Intern Med J 2015;45:702–10.

61. Woo SB, Lin D. Morsicatio Mucosae oris—a chronic oral frictional keratosis, not a leukoplakia. J Oral Maxillofac Surg 2009;67:140–6.

62. Natarajan E, Woo SB. Benign alveolar ridge keratosis (oral lichen simplex chronicus): A distinct clinicopathologic entity. J Am Acad Dermatol 2008; 58(1):151–7.

63. Woo SB. Oral pathology: a comprehensive atlas and text. Philadelphia: Elsevier; 2012.

64. van der Wal JE. Smoker's keratosis. Encyclopedia of pathology. Cham: Springer; 2018.

65. Rodu B, Jansson C. Smokeless tobacco and oral cancer: a review of the risks and determinants. Crit Rev Oral Biol Med 2004;15(5):252–63.

66. Warnakulasuriya KA, Ralhan R. Clinical, pathological, cellular and molecular lesions caused by oral smokeless tobacco–a review. J Oral Pathol Med 2007;36:63–77.

67. Neville BW, Day TA. Oral cancer and precancerous lesions. CA Cancer J Clin 2002;52:195–215.

68. Mortazavi H, Safi Y, Baharvand M, et al. Peripheral exophytic oral lesions: a clinical decision tree. Int J Dent 2017;2017:9193831.

69. Mortazavi H, Safi Y, Baharvand M, et al. Oral white lesions: an updated clinical diagnostic decision tree. Dent J (Basel) 2019;7(1):15.

70. Jiang M, Bu W, Chen X, et al. A case of irritation fibroma. Adv Dermatol Allergol 2019;36(1):125–6.

71. Sobhan M, Alirezaei P, Farshchian M, et al. White sponge nevus: report of a case and review of the literature. Acta Med Iran 2017;55(8):533–5.

72. Akpan A, Morgan R. Oral candidiasis. Postgrad Med J 2002;78:455–9.

73. Farah CS, Lynch N, McCullough MJ. Oral fungal infections: an update for the general practitioner. Aust Dent J 2010;55(1 Suppl):48–54.

74. Lewis MAO, Williams DW. Diagnosis and management of oral candidosis. Br Dent J 2017;223(9):675–81.

75. Tumban E. A current update on human papillomavirus-associated head and neck cancers. Viruses 2019;11(10):922.

76. Van Heerden WFP, Raubenheimer EJ, Bunn BK. Human papillomavirus infection of the oral cavity: what the dentist should know. SADJ 2017;17(2):52–5.

77. Bloem P, Ogbuanu I. Vaccination to prevent human papillomavirus infections: From promise to practice. PLoS Med 2017;14(6):e1002325.

78. Laprise JF, Chesson HW, Markowitz LE, et al. Effectiveness and cost-effectiveness of human papillomavirus vaccination through age 45 years in the United States. Ann Intern Med 2020;172(1):22–9.

Oral Hypersensitivity Reactions

Jacob P. Reinhart, MD[a],*, Eric T. Stoopler, DMD, FDSRCS, FDSRCPS[b], Glen H. Crawford, MD[c]

KEYWORDS

- Hypersensitivity reaction • Allergic contact stomatitis • Oral mucosa • Dental restorations
- Patch testing • Oral lichenoid reactions

KEY POINTS

- Oral hypersensitivity reactions are relatively uncommon when compared with cutaneous hypersensitivity reactions, owing in large part to the specific immunologic properties of the oral mucosa.
- Diagnosing oral hypersensitivity reactions relies on a detailed history and physical examination. A mucosal biopsy may also be performed to rule out other diagnoses.
- Patch testing is the gold standard for diagnosing allergic contact dermatitis on the skin.
- Patch testing is often used to evaluate patients suspected of having oral hypersensitivity reactions to dental materials, flavoring agents, and/or preservatives.
- Treatment of oral hypersensitivity reactions involves patient education, removal and/or avoidance of the implicated allergen, and/or use of topical corticosteroids for management.

INTRODUCTION

Although quite common on the skin, allergic contact hypersensitivity reactions on the oral mucosa are less commonly encountered in clinical practice. The term allergic contact dermatitis (ACD) is used when this reaction occurs on the skin and suggests relatively consistent physical and histopathologic features. The workup for ACD is often aided by the performance of epicutaneous patch testing. Oral hypersensitivity reactions (OHRs) involving the mucosa of the lips and mouth, however, often pose a more difficult diagnostic and therapeutic challenge. Clinical presentations of OHR are more varied; histopathologic findings are often ambiguous, and the strength of evidence for the use of epicutaneous patch testing is less robust than for ACD.

When present, physical signs of OHR can include erythema, ulceration, and lichenification. Symptoms of OHR can include burning, pain, itching, and paresthesias. Many of these signs and symptoms overlap with other inflammatory mucosal conditions, making their evaluation and management difficult. Despite these challenges, several conditions of the lips and oral mucosa are associated with oral hypersensitivity pathogenesis, including oral lichenoid reactions (OLRs) and allergic contact cheilitis.

In situations where these conditions are resistant to therapy or when the timing of onset correlates with a potential chemical exposure, referral to a patch test specialist may be indicated. The list of potential allergenic chemicals is vast; however, **Fig. 1** shows that allergens in OHR can be broadly categorized into dental materials (eg, dental metals, adhesives, and resins), flavorings, and preservatives (from food and oral hygiene products).

PATHOPHYSIOLOGY

Similar to ACD, the pathophysiology of OHR is a delayed type hypersensitivity, mediated primarily

[a] U.S. Navy, San Diego, CA, USA; [b] Department of Oral Medicine, University of Pennsylvania, Penn Dental Medicine, 240 South 40th Street, Room 206, Schattner Building, Philadelphia, PA 19104, USA; [c] Department of Dermatology, University of Pennsylvania, 822 Pine Street Suite 2A, Philadelphia, PA 19107, USA
* Corresponding author. Penn Dental Medicine, 240 South 40th Street, Room 206, Schattner Building, Philadelphia, PA 19104.
E-mail address: Reinhart.jacob@gmail.com

Dermatol Clin 38 (2020) 467–476
https://doi.org/10.1016/j.det.2020.05.007
0733-8635/20/Published by Elsevier Inc.

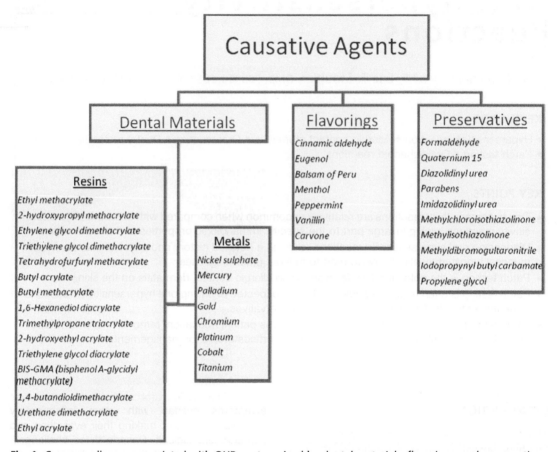

Fig. 1. Common allergens associated with OHRs, categorized by dental materials, flavorings, and preservatives.

by antigen-specific T-helper 1 cells. Allergic reactions only occur in individuals who were previously sensitized by contacting a specific allergen and subsequently developed this antigen-specific T-cell response, potentially even years after initial exposure. When an individual is reexposed to the allergen, a cell-mediated inflammatory response against basal keratinocytes is subsequently triggered, producing a wide array of physical inflammatory manifestations including edema, erythema, ulceration, and pruritus.

Despite daily exposure to a multitude of potential allergens and relatively direct access to mucosa-associated lymphoid tissue via increased tissue permeability and heavy oral vascularization, hypersensitivity responses to allergens occur less frequently in the oral cavity than on the skin.

One reason for the lower frequency of OHRs is oral mucosal tolerance. A number of complex regulatory mechanisms contribute to this process, including T-cell apoptosis and functional inactivation of T cells. These processes are specific to the oral mucosa and can influence an individual's systemic physiologic tolerance to an antigen. For example, it has been shown that young individuals exposed orally to nickel (ie, braces) have a higher likelihood of developing tolerance to nickel, whereas cutaneous ear piercing strongly favors sensitization to nickel when occurring before oral nickel exposure.[1]

Another physiologic mechanism that inhibits contact allergies is the rapid dilution of allergens from food and oral hygiene products by saliva and consumption of liquids. Allergens promptly migrate distally in the gastrointestinal tract, greatly decreasing the duration of contact with oral mucosa. Patients who have developed oral contact allergies often require prolonged intimate contact or repetitive interactions over many years.[2] Accordingly, the literature suggests the mean age of OLRs, a common hypersensitivity manifestation, to be 54.6 years of age.[3]

PATCH TESTING
Indications

Patch testing is the gold standard diagnostic method for detecting relevant contact allergens of the skin.[4] The methodology is based on demonstrating a delayed (type IV) cell-mediated hypersensitivity reaction by testing a series of potential allergens against a patient's skin, eliciting a delayed inflammatory reaction. Although the evidence for widespread use in the evaluation of all patients with OHR is questionable, patch testing in certain OHR scenarios can be useful.[5-7]

Patch testing in OHR is indicated when the history and physical findings raise the provider's suspicion for an allergic cause. However, the decision to refer to a patch test specialist should also consider the costs, time commitment for the patient, and geographic limitations of tertiary patch test referral centers.

Technique

In a standard patch test, a series of allergens are individually prepared in chamber wells and subsequently adhered as patches to a patient's unaffected skin, most commonly the upper back (**Fig. 2**A, B). The patches are secured under occlusion and individual chamber wells are marked on the skin to identify each tested allergen. After 48 hours of contact, the patches are removed, and a trained clinician interprets each positive reaction for clinical relevance (**Fig. 2**C). Readings are often repeated at 96 hours to allow for delayed presentations and for transient erythema to resolve.

Allergen Selection

More than 4000 different chemicals have been reported in the scientific literature to potentially cause hypersensitivity reactions.[4] The patch test specialist must use pretest probability assessment to select appropriate chemicals for patch testing. The Thin-layer Rapid Use Epicutaneous Test is the only series approved by the US Food and Drug Administration in the United States, currently consisting of 35 allergens and 1 control (**Fig. 3**). This commercially available test kit has increased the accessibility of patch testing to clinics and

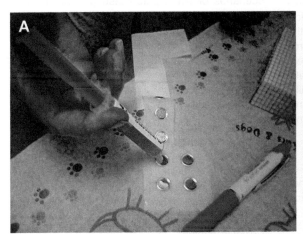
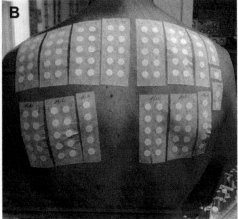
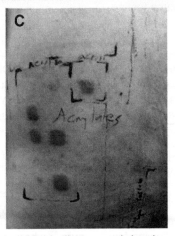

Fig. 2. Patch testing procedures require individually prepared chamber wells to be filled with selected allergens (A) and adhered as patches to a patient's unaffected skin, most commonly the upper back (B). After 48 to 96 hours, patches are removed to identify positive reactions (C).

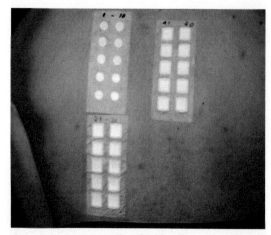

Fig. 3. The Thin-layer Rapid Use Epicutaneous (T.R.U.E.) Test is a US Food and Drug Administration–approved standard patch test kit with preselected allergens.

patients. However, as an abbreviated series, it may miss up to 27% of relevant allergens.[8] Consequently, patch test specialists typically select additional panels of allergens for testing based on the clinical situation and exposure history. For patients with oral disease, a patch test provider may select panels that include flavoring agents, dental metals, acrylates, and/or preservatives. Additionally, testing might include the patient's own personal care or oral hygiene products such as face creams, make-ups, lip balms, or dentifrices.

When to Involve a Patch Test Specialist

After limited (eg, Thin-layer Rapid Use Epicutaneous) patch testing, if there is still a strong suspicion for allergic causation, it would be reasonable to refer the patient to a tertiary patch test center for more expanded exposure-targeted patch testing.

Contraindications

A recent history of sun exposure may produce false-negative reactions because ultraviolet light can suppress local skin immune reactivity. The use of cutaneous topical corticosteroid creams and oral corticosteroids may suppress positive reactions. Patients taking other immunosuppressive agents may still undergo patch testing if discontinuing their medication is unavoidable.[9] Patch testing is not approved during pregnancy.

Determining the Relevance of Positive Reactions

The patch testing provider uses the following factors to formulate an opinion about clinical relevance: timing, distribution and morphology,

histopathologic features, patient exposure to known allergens, improvement after avoidance, worsening upon reexposure, exclusion of other diagnoses, and confirmatory patch test results.

LYMPHOCYTE TRANSFORMATION TESTING

In lymphocyte transformation testing (LTT), peripheral blood lymphocytes are tested in vitro against various antigens. After 7 days of incubation, the patient's sample is analyzed for proliferation of hapten-specific T cells, indicating a history of sensitization to the corresponding agent. Although less commonly used than patch testing, LTT has the advantage of being a simple blood test as compared with the inconvenience of several clinic visits and physical restrictions imposed during the patch test process over 4 or 5 days.

Limitations of LTTs include increased cost, paucity of qualified laboratories, and a limited number of haptens available for testing.[10] Despite these factors, LTTs may be used in some clinical scenarios or when patch testing is not feasible. LTT typically includes titanium, nickel, and mercury.[11] Some laboratories are able to test additional dental allergens such as aluminum, chromium, copper, gold, silver, tin, bone cement liquid and particles, and cobalt alloy particles.[11]

CLINICAL MANIFESTATIONS

Clinical manifestations of OHRs vary widely. Patients may endorse subjective symptoms of pain, burning sensation, paresthesia, and/or itching, sometimes without any overt clinical signs.[12] These reported symptoms may be suggestive of burning mouth syndrome, which is a separate and distinct clinical disorder not related to OHRs. Physical findings may include edema, erythema, lichenification, desquamation, vesicles, bullae, erosions, ulcers, and plaques.[12] The lack of specific or characteristic clinical presentation further complicates the evaluation and management of patients with OHR. Additionally, oral lesions and mucosal findings may be multifactorial in etiology with delayed hypersensitivity playing only a supporting role. Highlighted are the most common clinical entities associated with OHRs.

Oral Lichenoid Reactions

OLRs and oral lichen planus (OLP) have similar clinical and histopathologic features. They are differentiated by causality, with OLRs representing a reaction to an internal or external chemical exposure,[13] whereas OLP is an idiopathic inflammatory disorder.[14] OLRs are confined to the oral mucosa, whereas OLP is often associated with other cutaneous findings of lichen planus, such as flat-topped polygonal violaceous papules and plaques on the wrists, ankles, and genitalia.

Common locations of OLRs are the buccal mucosa or lateral borders of the tongue, often occurring unilaterally. Both OLRs and OLP present clinically as reticular white patches and plaques in the oral mucosa and have the potential for mucosal erosion (**Fig. 4**).[2] It should be noted, however, that some authors do not clinically differentiate the two diagnoses.[15]

Histologically, OLRs and OLP are indistinguishable. Inflammatory cell infiltration in the connective tissue with or without extension into the epithelium can be visualized.[2] Atrophic and orthokeratinized epithelium, often with a loss of a well-defined basal cell layer, along with keratinocyte apoptosis is characteristic.[16]

The literature supports contact hypersensitivity as one mechanism for the development of OLRs, with 60% to 80% of patients testing positive on patch testing.[5,17] Allergic causation is more common when the oral lichenoid lesions are in direct contact with or near the suspected dental restoration material.[18] The mercury constituent of dental amalgam is the most commonly reported allergen in OLRs. Other reported causal allergens include dental metals such as copper sulfate, nickel, palladium, and gold[2,19] and nonmetals such as resins, carvone, potassium dicyanoaurate, and balsam of Peru.[6,19]

Patch testing is recommended in patients with OLRs and a suspected allergic basis to their dental restorations.[19] Results may be helpful in selecting materials for future dental procedures. Additionally, patch test reactions may be used as part of the risk/benefit analysis in deciding whether to remove a restoration. There are conflicting reports in the literature regarding the potential benefit of removing amalgam and/or dental restorations in the setting of positive patch test reactions. Without removal, patients may improve with directed therapy over time. Some reports have indicated that patients may not improve after removal.[20] Others have demonstrated that removal of restorations results in improvement in 35% to 100% of patients and complete resolution in 33%.[18,21] Improvement may be early as a few days[22] to 3 months[18] and is more likely in lesions located directly adjacent to dental amalgam.[23]

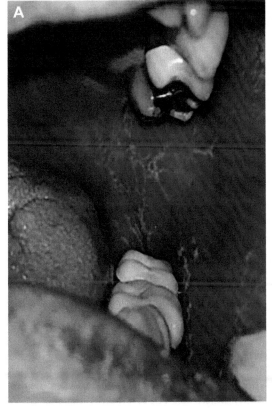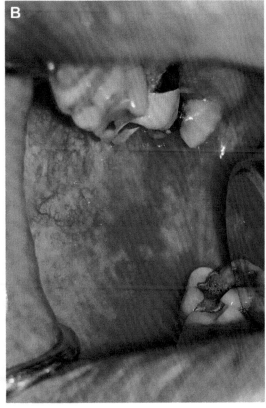

Fig. 4. Visual comparison of (*A*) reticular OLP affecting the left buccal mucosa and (*B*) OLR affecting the right buccal mucosa.

Allergic Contact Cheilitis

Cheilitis is a relatively common dermatologic condition characterized by inflammation of the lips, vermillion border, and surrounding tissue (**Fig. 5**). Symptoms include pain, fissuring, and edema. Simple cheilitis may result from xerosis or from irritant exposures, but allergic contact reactions may play a significant role in refractory cases of cheilitis.[24] Of patients presenting with cheilitis, 25% to 85% may have positive patch testing reactions, with 20% to 65% of those being clinically relevant.[6,25]

The most common allergens affecting patients with allergic contact cheilitis are fragrances, oral hygiene products, and food preservatives, to include balsam of Peru, benzoate, and dodecyl gallate.[6,25,26] As such, patients with suspected allergic contact cheilitis should be patch tested with a series of preservatives and flavorings.[6] After identification of implicating allergens, patients with allergic contact cheilitis should avoid continued exposures.

CAUSATIVE AGENTS
Dental Materials

Materials used in dentistry restorations (crowns, bridges, fillings, etc) contain several constituent chemicals that may cause hypersensitivity reactions of the oral mucosa. The most common constituent chemicals include metals (eg, nickel, mercury, chromium, palladium, and gold) and resins (eg, acrylate monomers and polymers). When lesions are localized to mucosal sites adjacent to dental restorations, the likelihood of allergenic cause is amplified.[7]

Approximately 14% of patients with a suspected hypersensitivity reaction to their dental restorations were found to have relevant patch testing

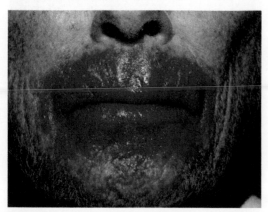

Fig. 5. A prominent display of allergic contact cheilitis in response to topical corticosteroids.

to dental materials, with metals being the most common triggers.[27] One study showed that common metal allergens with positive reactions on patch testing included gold (14.0%), nickel sulfate (13.2%), mercury (9.9%), palladium chloride (7.4%), and cobalt chloride (5.0%).[7] Despite these results, it is estimated that sensitization to gold and nickel often occurs from sources other than dental agents.[7] **Fig. 1** lists dental material allergens (metals, resins), the most common of which are detailed in the next section.

Metals

Nickel sulfate is one of the most commonly used metals in dental alloys owing to its favorable mechanical properties and relatively low cost. Unfortunately, it is also the most common sensitizer among all metals.[28] The North American Contact Dermatitis Group patch tested 5085 adults and found that 19.5% had a positive reaction to nickel.[29] It has been postulated that up to 20% of cases of nickel sensitization are the result of exposure to alloys in dental restorations.[30]

In comparison with the high prevalence of nickel sensitivity in the general population, OHRs attributed to nickel are much less frequent. When confirmed, nickel hypersensitivity in the oral mucosa may present with OLRs, gingival hyperplasia, burnings sensation, or lingual paresthesia.

In individuals with positive patch testing to nickel and compelling clinical features of an OHR to dental nickel, a replacement with stainless steel or titanium molybdenum alloy may be considered.[31] Despite a small amount of nickel present in stainless steel alloy, orthodontic appliances made from stainless steel do not tend to initiate hypersensitivity reactions.[32]

Mercury is used in the making of dental amalgam, an alloy that has long been used for dental restorations. In addition to silver, tin, and copper, liquid mercury is mixed to produce the dental amalgam.[2] Hypersensitivity reactions to dental amalgam typically manifest as OLRs localized to the tissue adjacent to dental restorations.[33] It has been postulated that, over time, saliva can release mercury from the amalgam in the form of vapor or salt.[13] This release is augmented with everyday processes such as chewing, eating, and drinking. Complicating the assessment of patients with potential oral hypersensitivity to dental amalgam is the high rate of false-positive patch test reactions. Currently available patch tests to mercury use dilute solutions of corrosive mercury salts, which can cause irritant reactions on the skin and can be misinterpreted as a positive reaction.[34,35]

Although previously thought to be an unlikely cause of OHR,[36] the more recent introduction of the salt disodium tetrachloropalladate as a patch test allergen has substantially increased the diagnosis of palladium sensitivity.[37] Palladium OHRs have been associated with oral lichenoid lesions, metallic taste, and xerostomia.[37] The frequency of lichenoid reactions ranges from 13% to 15% among individuals with a documented palladium sensitivity.[38]

Although perhaps decreasing in use in the United States, gold remains an important dental metal in global populations.[39,40] In patients undergoing patch testing to dental series, 25% to 30% demonstrate positive reactions to gold salts; however, the clinical relevance of these somewhat frequent positive reactions is often difficult to ascertain.[39,40] Clinical improvements from the removal of gold-containing dental appliances in individuals with a documented contact allergy to gold are limited to small populations of individuals and case reports in the literature.[39,41,42] Gold dental crowns are, however, correlated with orofacial granulomatosis,[43] with the area of exposed gold surfaces in the oral cavity correlating positively with the extent of allergic reaction.[40] Although it should still be considered as a possible cause of allergic contact stomatitis or OLRs,[41] it has been suggested that an overrepresentation of gold allergies in individuals with gold-containing dental appliances exists.[39]

Resins, Acrylates, and Other Dental Materials

In addition to metals, composite resins used in dental restorations may produce OLRs or other symptoms after contacting the lips or oral mucosa (see **Fig. 1**).[43] Acrylic dental adhesive agents used with metal braces have been reported to cause OHRs with successful symptomatic resolution after removal of the braces.[44] Positive patch testing has been identified to mixed polyether impression materials, base paste, catalyst paste, and base component, suggesting a possible hypersensitivity etiology (see **Fig. 2**C).[45,46] This finding underscores the importance of patch testing using a comprehensive series for dental adhesives and acrylates.

Substitution and/or replacement of dental materials is an expensive and invasive process that should be only considered if the following parameters are met[47]:

1. A temporal association has been established between the suspected dental material and onset of clinical signs and/or symptoms,
2. Objective clinical examination findings support the aforementioned association, and

3. Challenge testing confirms a reaction to the suspected dental material.

Hygiene Products

Hygiene products can contain many flavorings agents and preservatives capable of causing oral allergic reactions. A thorough history should be taken from patients with suspected OHRs to uncover exposure to potentially allergenic components in these products. For example, cheilitis has been reported as a contact allergy to the rubber on a modern toothbrush[48] as well as stannous fluoride (tin [II] fluoride) in toothpaste.[49]

Flavoring Agents

Flavoring agents found in food, cosmetics, and oral hygiene products have the potential to generate hypersensitivity reactions. Patients with oral symptoms suggestive of hypersensitivity reactions may test positive to a number of flavoring agents (see **Fig. 1**). When patients are found to have positive patch test reactions and clinical symptoms consistent with OHR, recommendations can be made for alternative hygiene products without the implicated allergenic constituents.

Cinnamic aldehyde is a widely used flavoring agent present in mouthwash, lip balm, chewing gum, candy, and toothpaste. Reports of intraoral ACD to cinnamic aldehyde are limited but do exist.[50,51] Patch test data are also restricted because it is often not tested outside of its presence in fragrance mix I.[6,52] Clinical presentation of intraoral and perioral reactions varies widely, but can be classified under contact stomatitis.[50] Owing to its high prevalence within the consumer market, a high index of suspicion is required to effectively diagnosis this condition.[50]

Eugenol is a commonly used flavoring agent extracted from spices like cloves and cinnamon.[53] In addition to cinnamic aldehyde, it constitutes another 1 of the 8 components in the commonly tested fragrance mix. Eugenol can also be used in dental restorations, or as an anesthetic or antimicrobial agent.[54] When tested as a single allergen, eugenol has been showed to elicit positive reactions in 0% to 2% of patients with oral symptoms.[5,6] Case reports have identified eugenol allergies producing aphthous stomatitis, allergic contact gingivitis, and symptoms of burning mouth from chemical trauma.[53,55,56]

Balsam of Peru is the balsam or resin obtained from tree bark of the *Myroxylon pereirae*. It is found in foods, cosmetics (lip balm) and personal hygiene products (toothpaste and mouthwash).[57] In one study, it was the second most common flavoring agent (behind fragrance mix) to elicit positive reactions on patch testing (7.2% of patients with oral symptoms).[6] In addition, the pooled prevalence of sensitization to balsam of Peru in the general population is 1.8%.[58]

Peppermint oil, or *Mentha piperita* oil, is another flavoring agent commonly found in cosmetic and personal hygiene products. Its role in OHRs is limited to case reports in the literature.[59,60] One study showed that 0.7% of patients with oral symptoms had positive reactions to peppermint oil.[6] Nevertheless, peppermint oil should be strongly considered as an allergen in patients with oral symptoms and/or perioral dermatitis.

Preservatives

Preservatives are also a common cause of OHRs. The most common preservative allergens are listed in **Fig 1**.

Management

It is advisable for patients to eliminate suspected flavoring agents and/or oral hygiene products for a brief period (approximately 4–6 weeks according to authors opinion) to determine if they are potential sources of hypersensitivity reactions. If the reaction resolves after the elimination period, the patient may reintroduce a single eliminated product every 5 to 7 days (in these authors' opinion) to identify the specific trigger(s) and avoid them in future. If the reaction persists after the elimination period, clinicians can consider tissue biopsy to aid in diagnosis and rule out other conditions with similar clinical appearances (eg, OLP). If the trigger for the reaction is not identified, topical corticosteroids, such as triamcinolone paste 0.1% or fluocinonide gel 0.05%, may applied to the affected area(s) for symptom management.

SUMMARY

With numerous potential allergens, overlapping symptoms and presentation, and challenges of diagnostic workup, the management of OHRs can present a formidable challenge. Effective diagnosis and management of hypersensitivity reactions requires skilled clinical evaluation. Clinicians should acquire a detailed history of the patient's specific concerns to include onset and time course of oral symptoms. Patients with a history suspicious for hypersensitivity etiology should be considered for patch testing.

Patch testing can be useful, but is not always diagnostic. After identifying relevant allergens from patch testing, treatment of OHRs is centered on avoidance. This process that can be challenging and even unattainable for some patients,

particularly with respect to dental restorations. If patients can successfully avoid triggering allergens, symptom improvement and resolution can be achieved.

Future research should aim to support and identify patients with hypersensitivity reactions, and also aim to delineate specific hypersensitivity components of existing oral conditions.

DISCLOSURE

The authors have nothing to disclose.

REFERENCES

1. Van Hoogstraten IM, Andersen KE, Von Blomberg BM, et al. Reduced frequency of nickel allergy upon oral nickel contact at an early age. Clin Exp Immunol 1991;85:441–5.
2. McParland H, Warnakulasuriya S. Oral lichenoid contact lesions to mercury and dental amalgam—a review. J Biomed Biotechnol 2012;2012:589569.
3. Thornhill MH, Pemberton MN, Simmons RK, et al. Amalgam-contact hypersensitivity lesions and oral lichen planus. Oral Surg Oral Med Oral Pathol Oral Radiol Endod 2003;95(3):291–9.
4. Mowad CM, Anderson B, Scheinman P, et al. Allergic contact dermatitis: patient diagnosis and evaluation. J Am Acad Dermatol 2016;74:1029–40.
5. Kim TW, Kim WI, Mun JH, et al. Patch testing with dental screening series in oral disease. Ann Dermatol 2015;27:389–93.
6. Torgerson RR, Davis MD, Bruce AJ, et al. Contact allergy in oral disease. J Am Acad Dermatol 2007;57:315–21.
7. Khamaysi Z, Bergman R, Weltfriend S. Positive patch test reactions to allergens of the dental series and the relation to the clinical presentations. Contact Dermatitis 2006;55(4):216–8.
8. Warshaw EM, Belsito DV, Taylor JS, et al. North American Contact Dermatitis Group. Patch test results for 2009-2010. Dermatitis 2013;24:50–9.
9. Wee JS, White JM, McFadden JP, et al. Patch testing in patients treated with systemic immunosuppression and cytokine inhibitors. Contact Dermatitis 2010;62:165–9.
10. Crawford GH. The role of patch testing in the evaluation of orthopedic implant-related adverse effects: current evidence does not support broad use. Dermatitis 2013;24:99–103.
11. MELISA. Allergens tested. 2019. Available at: http://www.vin.com/Members/Proceedings/. Accessed March 1, 2020.
12. Tosti A, Piraccini BM, Peluso AM. Contact and irritant stomatitis. Semin Cutan Med Surg 1997;16:314–9.
13. Minciullo PL, Paolino G, Vacca M, et al. Unmet diagnostic needs in contact oral mucosal allergies. Clin Mol Allergy 2016;14(1):10.

14. Kamath VV, Setlur K, Yerlagudda K. Oral lichenoid lesions—a review and update. Indian J Dermatol 2015;60:102.

15. Yiannias JA, El-Azhary RA, Hand JH, et al. Relevant contact sensitivities in patients with the diagnosis of oral lichen planus. J Am Acad Dermatol 2000;42(2): 177–82.

16. Schiodt M. Oral discoid lupus erythematosus. III. A histopathologic study of sixty-six patients. Oral Surg Oral Med Oral Pathol 1984;57(3):281–93.

17. Suter VG, Warnakulasuriya S. The role of patch testing in the management of oral lichenoid reactions. J Oral Pathol Med 2016;45:48–57.

18. Thanyavuthi A, Boonchai W, Kasemsarn P. Amalgam contact allergy in oral lichenoid lesions. Dermatitis 2016;27:215–21.

19. Ahlgren C, Axell T, Moller H, et al. Contact allergies to potential allergens in patients with oral lichen lesions. Clin Oral Investig 2014;18:227–37.

20. Ostman PO, Anneroth G, Skoglund A. Amalgam-associated oral lichenoid reactions. Clinical and histologic changes after removal of amalgam fillings. Oral Surg Oral Med Oral Pathol Oral Radiol Endod 1996;81:459–65.

21. Koch P, Bahmer FA. Oral lesions and symptoms related to metals used in dental restorations: a clinical, allergological, and histologic study. J Am Acad Dermatol 1999;41:422–30.

22. Smart ER, Macleod RI, Lawrence CM. Resolution of lichen planus following removal of amalgam restorations in patients with proven allergy to mercury salts: a pilot study. Br Dent J 1995;178(3):108–12.

23. Issa Y, Brunton PA, Glenny AM, et al. Healing of oral lichenoid lesions after replacing amalgam restorations: a systematic review. Oral Surg Oral Med Oral Pathol Oral Radiol Endod 2004;98:553–65.

24. Kohorst JJ, Bruce AJ, Torgerson RR. Mucosal lesions in an allergy practice. Curr Allergy Asthma Rep 2016;16:26.

25. Schena D, Fantuzzi F, Girolomoni G. Contact allergy in chronic eczematous lip dermatitis. Eur J Dermatol 2008;18:688–92.

26. Rosen A, Ngshanyi S, Tosti A, et al. Allergic contact cheilitis in children and improvement with patch testing. JAAD Case Rep 2016;26:25–8.

27. Mittermuller P, Hiller KA, Schmalz G, et al. Five hundred patients reporting on adverse effects from dental materials: frequencies, complaints, symptoms, allergies. Dent Mater 2018;34:1756–68.

28. Covington JS, McBride MA, Slagle WF, et al. Quantization of nickel and beryllium leakage from base metal alloys. J Prosthet Dent 1989;54(1):127–36.

29. Fransway AF, Zug KA, Belsito DV, et al. North American Contact Dermatitis Group patch test results for 2007-2008. Dermatitis 2013;24:10–21.

30. Imirzalioglu P, Alaaddinoglu E, Yilmaz Z, et al. Influence of recasting different types of dental alloys on gingival fibroblast cytotoxicity. J Prosthet Dent 2012; 107:24–33.

31. Noble J, Ahing SI, Karaiskos NE, et al. Nickel allergy and orthodontics, a review and report of two cases. Br Dent J 2008;204:297–300.

32. Jensen CS, Lisby S, Baadsgaard O, et al. Release of nickel ions from stainless steel alloys used in dental braces and their patch test reactivity in nickel-sensitive individuals. Contact Dermatitis 2003;48(6):300–4.

33. Duxbury AJ, Watts DC, Ead RD. Allergy to dental amalgam. Br Dent J 1982;152:344.

34. National Council Against Health Fraud. Position paper on amalgam fillings. 2002. Available at: http://www.ncahf.org. Accessed July 13, 2019.

35. Fisher AA. The misuse of patch test to determine 'hypersensitivity' to mercury amalgam dental fillings. Cutis 1985;35(109):112–7.

36. Wataha JC, Hanks CT. Biological effects of palladium and risk of using palladium in dental casting alloys. J Oral Rehabil 1996;23:309–20.

37. Muris J, Goossens A, Goncalo M, et al. Sensitization to palladium and nickel in Europe and the relationship with oral disease and dental alloys. Contact Dermatitis 2015;72:286–96.

38. Durosaro O, el-Azhary RA. A 10-year retrospective study on palladium sensitivity. Dermatitis 2009;20:208–13.

39. Vamnes JS, Morken T, Helland S, et al. Dental gold alloys and contact hypersensitivity. Contact Dermatitis 2000;42:128–33.

40. Ahlgren C, Ahnlide I, Björkner B, et al. Contact allergy to gold is correlated to dental gold. Acta Derm Venereol 2002;82:41–4.

41. Laeijendecker R, van Joost T. Oral manifestations of gold allergy. J Am Acad Dermatol 1994;30:205–9.

42. Lazarov A, Kidron D, Tulchinsky Z, et al. Contact orofacial granulomatosis caused by delayed hypersensitivity to gold and mercury. J Am Acad Dermatol 2003;49:1117–20.

43. Blomgren J, Axéll T, Sandahl O, et al. Adverse reactions in the oral mucosa associated with anterior composite restorations. J Oral Pathol Med 1996; 25(6):311–3.

44. Kiviat J, Fleming Y. Orthodontic appliance intolerance due to dental adhesive allergy. Dermatitis 2018;29:349–50.

45. Batchelor JM, Todd PM. Allergic contact stomatitis caused by a polyether dental impression material. Contact Dermatitis 2010;63(5):296–7.

46. Mittermuller P, Szeimies RM, Landthaler M, et al. A rare allergy to a polyether dental impression material. Clin Oral Investig 2012;16(4):1111–6.

47. Stoopler ET, De Rossi SS. AAOM clinical practice statement: subject: oral contact allergy. Oral Surg Oral Med Oral Pathol Oral Radiol 2016;122(1):50–2.

48. Harris V, Smith S. Don't brush off contact allergies in cheilitis: modern toothbrush contact dermatitis. J Am Acad Dermatol 2017;76(suppl):AB103.

49. Enamandram M, Das S, Chaney KS. Cheilitis and urticaria associated with stannous fluoride in toothpaste. J Am Acad Dermatol 2014;71:e75–6.

50. Isaac-Renton M, Li MK, Parsons LM. Cinnamon spice and everything not nice: many features of intraoral allergy to cinnamic aldehyde. Dermatitis 2015;26:116–21.

51. Calapai G, Miroddi M, Mannucci C, et al. Oral adverse reactions due to cinnamon-flavoured chewing gums consumption. Oral Dis 2014;20:637–43.

52. Shah M, Lewis FM, Gawkrodger DJ. Contact allergy in patients with oral symptoms: a study of 47 patients. Am J Contact Dermat 1996;7:146–51.

53. Navarro Trivino FJ, Cuenca-Barralex C, Ruiz-Villaverde R. Eugenol allergy mimicking recurrent aphthous stomatitis and burning mouth syndrome. Contact Dermatitis 2019;81(6):462–3.

54. Marchese A, Barbieri R, Coppo E, et al. Antimicrobial activity of eugenol and essential oils containing eugenol: a mechanistic viewpoint. Crit Rev Microbiol 2017;43:668–89.

55. Silvestre JF, Albares M, Blanes M, et al. Allergic contact gingivitis due to eugenol present in a restorative dental material. Contact Dermatitis 2005;52:341.

56. Bui TNPT, Mose KF, Anersen F. Eugenol allergy mimicking burning mouth syndrome. Contact Dermatitis 2016;80:54–5.

57. LeSueur BW, Yiannias JA. Contact stomatitis. Dermatol Clin 2003;21:105–14.

58. Alinaghi F, Bennike NH, Egeberg A, et al. Prevalence of contact allergy in the general population: a systematic review and meta-analysis. Contact Dermatitis 2019;80:77–85.

59. Morton C, Garioch J, Todd P, et al. Contact sensitivity to menthol and peppermint in patients with intra-oral symptoms. Contact Dermatitis 1995;32:281–4.

60. Herro E, Jacob SE. Menthapiperita (peppermint). Dermatitis 2010;21:327–9.

Burning Mouth Syndrome

Brittany Klein, DDS[a], Jaisri R. Thoppay, DDS, MBA, MS[b],
Scott S. De Rossi, DMD, MBA[c], Katharine Ciarrocca, DMD, MSEd[d],*

KEYWORDS

• Oral burning • Dry mouth • Glossodynia • Burning mouth syndrome • Oral dysesthesia

KEY POINTS

• Burning mouth syndrome (BMS) is a chronic condition characterized by a burning sensation of the intraoral mucosa in the absence of a local or systemic cause.
• A diagnosis of BMS should be made only after a thorough history, clinical examination, and indicated laboratory studies have ruled out local or systemic cause.
• Despite advances in the understanding and treatment of BMS, it remains a challenging condition for both patients and providers.
• Some patients experience at least partial remission of symptoms with or without treatment, but, for many, symptoms persist. Management should be aimed at symptom reduction and coping strategies.

INTRODUCTION

Burning mouth syndrome (BMS) is a chronic condition characterized by a burning sensation of the intraoral mucosa in the absence of a local or systemic cause.[1–3] It is primarily a diagnosis of exclusion based on subjective symptoms.[4–6] The International Classification of Headache Disorders, Third Edition (ICHD-3), stipulates that, for a diagnosis of BMS, the burning sensation or dysesthesia must recur daily for more than 2 h/d for more than 3 months, without any clinically evident causative lesions.[7] The World Health Organization adds that BMS is characterized by significant emotional distress or interference with orofacial functions and lowers the symptom threshold to recurring for 2 h/d on 50% of the days for more than 3 months.[2]

The characteristic burning sensation of BMS is typically bilateral and is most commonly experienced on the tongue, although it can be experienced anywhere in the intraoral mucosa, including the lips, hard palate, gingiva, and buccal mucosa.[4,5,8] The sensation does not follow peripheral nerve distributions.[5] The onset of BMS is most often spontaneous and symptoms progress gradually in most patients, often persisting for several years.[8–10] Complete spontaneous resolution after 5 years has been reported in less than 3% of affected individuals, and less than 30% of patients with BMS show moderate symptom improvement with or without treatment.[9] The cause and pathophysiology of BMS are not well understood, although various mechanisms have been explored.[4,5,11] There is no known cure for BMS and management is aimed at symptom reduction. A variety of topical, systemic, and behavioral therapies have been used in the treatment of BMS with varied success.[4,12–14]

EPIDEMIOLOGY

BMS first appeared in the medical literature in the 1800s[15] and has also been referred to as burning mouth, oral dysesthesia, stomatodynia, glossodynia, and glossopyrosis.[2,5,6] There has historically been significant heterogeneity in the definition of BMS used in the literature, with several studies

[a] Division of Oral Medicine and Dentistry, Brigham and Women's Hospital, 1620 Tremont St, Suite 3-02B, Boston, MA 02120, USA; [b] Center for Integrative Oral Health Inc., 7151, University Boulevard, Unit 110, Winter Park, FL 32792, USA; [c] University of North Carolina-Chapel Hill, Adams School of Dentistry, Campus Box 7450, Chapel Hill, NC 27599-7450, USA; [d] University of North Carolina-Chapel Hill, Adams School of Dentistry, Chapel Hill, NC 27599-7450, USA
* Corresponding author.
E-mail address: kate_ciarrocca@unc.edu

Dermatol Clin 38 (2020) 477–483
https://doi.org/10.1016/j.det.2020.05.008

including patients whose burning sensation is attributable to an underlying condition.[2,3,12] Because of this, the estimated prevalence of BMS varies widely, with reports ranging from 0.7% to 8% of the population.[3,16] BMS has a strong female predilection, with women affected up to 7 times more than men.[8,10,13,16] Almost all patients with BMS are perimenopausal and postmenopausal women, with symptoms presenting between 3 years and 12 years following the onset of menopause.[3,4] The mean age at diagnosis is between 59 and 61 years, and BMS rarely occurs before the age of 30 years.[6,17]

CLASSIFICATION

BMS may be classified as primary or secondary.[13] In this model, primary BMS refers to a persistent burning sensation in the absence of clinical findings, and secondary BMS refers to a burning sensation related to an identifiable underlying condition. Consensus definitions have since moved away from this model in favor of stricter criteria in which burning sensation attributable to an underlying condition is not considered BMS.[2,7]

BMS can also be classified based on variations in pain intensity over a 24-hour period (**Fig. 1**). In

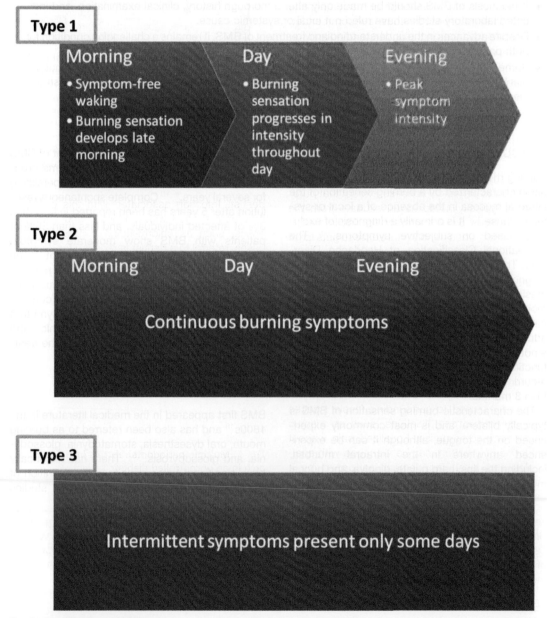

Fig. 1. Classification of BMS.

this model, type 1 BMS is characterized by symptom-free waking with burning sensation developing in the late morning, progressing throughout the day, and peaking in intensity in the evening. Type 2 BMS is the most common presentation and is characterized by continuous burning throughout the day, which makes falling asleep difficult. In type 3 BMS, patients have intermittent symptoms present only on some days.[8,18,19]

CAUSE AND PATHOPHYSIOLOGY

The cause of BMS is not well understood, but there is an emerging consensus that, for most patients, it is neuropathic.[4,5,7,11,20,21] BMS may represent a convergent clinical presentation of dysfunction arising in the peripheral nervous system, central nervous system, or both.[4,5]

It has been proposed that most BMS cases can be attributed to peripheral small fiber neuropathy in the intraoral mucosal epithelium.[5,20] Tongue biopsies performed in patients with BMS have revealed a decreased density of small fiber nerve endings compared with controls, consistent with a small fiber neuropathy, although these studies have been performed on a limited number of subjects and may not be generalizable to all patients with BMS.[5,22,23] Immunostaining of tongue biopsies has also revealed an increased expression of transient receptor potential cation channel subfamily V member 1 (TRPV1) channels.[24] TRP channels play an important role in temperature perception, sensitization, and nociception, and an increased number of TRPV1 receptors could contribute to a heightened pain sensation.[4,5,11]

Another subset of BMS may constitute a subclinical trigeminal neuropathy, a theory based on abnormalities of the masseter and blink reflexes, which are commonly evaluated when testing trigeminal nerve function, observed in approximately 20% of patients with BMS.[5] The remainder of patients may experience BMS as centrally mediated pain, possibly related to the hypofunction of dopaminergic neurons in the basal ganglia, which are involved in the inhibitory modulation of pain.[25] Alterations in this system are similar to those observed in Parkinson disease, and there is some evidence of an increased incidence of BMS in patients with Parkinson disease.[5] Decreased levels of dopamine in the basal ganglia of some patients with BMS may represent a common disease pathway for BMS and depression, which are often comormid.[5] Importantly, peripheral and central nervous system involvement are not mutually exclusive, nor are they clinically

differentiable without further testing. However, determining the underlying disorder in a given patient may allow more targeted therapy.[5,11]

CLINICAL FEATURES

BMS has a varied clinical presentation. The characteristic burning sensation is typically bilateral and is experienced most commonly on the tongue, followed by the anterior hard palate and labial mucosa.[8,16,17] Patients may describe this burning as scalding, tingling, or numb.[3,12,13] The reported intensity of pain experienced varies widely, but most patients describe their pain as mild or moderate on 0 to 10 numerical pain scales as well as on subjective descriptions of mild, moderate, and severe pain.[17] For some patients, the burning sensation is exacerbated by consuming hot foods or drinks and relieved by cold.[8,12,20] Xerostomia is a common complaint in patients with BMS.[16] Although there do not seem to be differences in stimulated saliva flow between patients with BMS and controls, there is some evidence of decreased unstimulated salivary flow and of different salivary composition.[26,27] However, these findings are controversial because hyposalivation represents an identifiable underlying cause, thus precluding patients with this presentation from a diagnosis of BMS.

Many patients with BMS experience taste disturbances, including persistent metallic or bitter taste and alterations in salty, sweet, or bitter tastes.[8,11] There is some evidence that BMS and taste dysfunction are linked via hypofunction, damage, or loss of inhibition to the chorda tympani, a branch of the facial nerve that caries taste sensation to the anterior two-thirds of the tongue.[11,28–30] Psychological and psychiatric factors have been found to play a role in BMS, with anxiety and depression being commonly observed comorbid conditions.[31] Sleep disturbances are also widely reported, including trouble falling asleep, awakening during the night, and poor sleep quality.[8,19,32]

DIFFERENTIAL DIAGNOSIS

BMS can be a debilitating, chronic condition, so it is imperative that local and systemic causative factors be ruled out. Local factors include parafunctional habits (eg, bruxism, tongue thrust) and poorly fitting dentures.[3,4,6,33] Each of these can produce microtrauma and local erythema that result in a burning sensation.[33] Clinical findings indicate that parafunctional habits include waking up with headaches, tenderness in the muscles of mastication on palpation, and partner observation of grinding at night.[6] Candidiasis, a common oral fungal infection produced by *Candida albicans*, is another common local cause of oral burning.[3,4,12,33] Geographic tongue, lichen planus, and other oral mucosal diseases should be ruled out via clinical examination.[6,12] Local allergic reactions, possibly to dental materials or to new toothpaste or mouthwashes, may also result in a burning sensation.[6,33,34] Systemic factors that can cause or exacerbate oral burning include medications, vitamin deficiencies, and systemic disease. Various medications have been shown to produce oral burning as a side effect, including antihistamines and antihypertensives, especially angiotensin-converting enzyme inhibitors, antiarrhythmics, and benzodiazpenes.[33] Several nutritional deficiencies have been explored in BMS, including vitamins B_{12}, B_6, D, iron, and zinc.[33] In addition, gastroesophageal reflux, diabetes mellitus, and hypothyroidism are diseases that can all cause oral burning[4,12,33] (**Fig. 2**).

Evaluation of a patient presenting with a complaint of oral burning should begin with a thorough history. The history of present illness, medications, allergies, medical history, a thorough review of systems, and recent dental procedures should all be reviewed to identify factors that may cause oral burning as well as any comorbid conditions. An extraoral examination (including gross cranial nerve assessment) and an intraoral examination should be performed, noting any changes in mucosal color, consistency, or texture. The examination should also include an evaluation of the dentition, periodontium, and any removable prostheses. Additional diagnostic work-up may include laboratory studies, as indicated, to rule out systemic conditions or nutritional deficiencies. Patch testing for allergens may also be helpful if

there are clinical signs of a hypersensitivity reaction, as well as fungal cultures if candidiasis is suspected and empiric therapy fails. Biopsy is not indicated to confirm a diagnosis of BMS[6] (**Fig. 3**).

MANAGEMENT

A variety of topical, systemic, and behavioral therapies have been used, with mixed results, in the treatment of BMS (**Table 1**). Clonazepam, a benzodiazepine that agonizes the inhibitory neurotransmitter gamma-aminobutyric acid (GABA), has been used both topically and systemically to manage BMS and has been shown to reduce symptoms in both short-term and long-term intervals.[3,4,6,14,35,36] Side effects of clonazepam include xerostomia, lethargy, and fatigue.[35] Importantly, clonazepam can cause physiologic and psychological dependence, whether used systemically or topically.[3] Patients should be made aware of this risk and advised to take the medication as prescribed and not to discontinue abruptly.

Capsaicin, a neuropeptide extracted from chili peppers that binds to TRPV1, can be applied topically to treat BMS through the proposed mechanism of reducing the number of TRPV1 receptors, leading to long-term desensitization of pain receptors to heat.[4,6,37,38] Although this method may cause increased burning immediately following application, it has been shown to produce long-term symptom relief.[14]

Alpha-lipoic acid (ALA), an antioxidant with a role in nerve repair, has been shown to improve BMS symptoms in some studies, but these results have been inconsistent and there has been considerable heterogeneity among trials.[3,6,14] There have been reports of increased heartburn, gastrointestinal upset, and headaches with ALA.

Local factors	Systemic factors	Psychologic Factors
• Poorly fitting dentures • Parafunctional habits • Candidiasis • Oral mucosal diseases • Local allergic reaction	• Nutritional deficiencies – Vitamin B12, B6, iron, zinc • Endocrine disorders – Diabetes mellitus, thyroid disease, hormonal deficiencies • Hyposalivation • Medication side effect • Upper respiratory tract infection • Gastroesophageal reflex disease	• Depression • Anxiety

Fig. 2. Factors associated with oral burning.

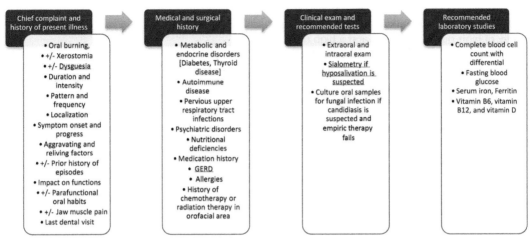

Fig. 3. Diagnostic work-up for BMS.

Although its use is less evidence based than some alternatives, ALA is offered by some clinicians as a first-line therapy, particularly for patients who wish to avoid prescription medications.[3]

Gabapentin is an anticonvulsant that has been successfully used to treat other neuropathic pain conditions. It has been shown to reduce symptoms in patients with BMS, especially when used in conjunction with ALA.[4,6,14]

Antidepressants, including tricyclic antidepressants (TCAs), selective serotonin reuptake inhibitors, and serotonin-norepinephrine reuptake inhibitors (SNRIs), have been explored as possible therapeutic agents for BMS.[3,4,6,14] Antidepressants have long been used in the management of neuropathic pain conditions.[39] TCAs, such as amitriptyline and nortriptyline, have been found to be most effective, but SNRIs, a newer class of antidepressant, are gaining

acceptance for pain relief. This acceptance is promising in the treatment of BMS because SNRIs are associated with fewer anticholinergic effects, including xerostomia, than TCAs.[39] The evidence on these medications in the treatment of BMS is limited, but, given the impact of BMS on quality of life and mood, they may benefit patients when prescribed and managed by a qualified practitioner.[3]

There is some evidence that cognitive behavior therapy (CBT) can be effective in managing patients with BMS, particularly resistant BMS.[3] In the context of BMS, CBT can help to reduce pain catastrophizing and to improve mood and coping strategies.[3,4] Long-term symptom improvement has also been observed.[4,14] Intraoral devices designed to mitigate parafunctional tongue habits have also shown limited benefit in BMS symptom management.[40]

Table 1
Pharmacotherapeutic interventions

Category	Medication	Topical or Systemic	Dose and Delivery
Benzodiazepine	Clonazepam	Topical	0.5 mg to 2 mg swish and expectorate or tablet held in mouth and expectorated
		Systemic	0.5 mg capsule or orally disintegrating tablet starting dose taken at bedtime, not to exceed 2mg/d
Tricyclic antidepressant	Amitriptyline	Systemic	10–25-mg starting dose taken at bedtime, titrated to maximum dose of 100–125 mg
Anticonvulsant	Gabapentin	Systemic	300 mg/d at bedtime starting dose, up to 900–1200 mg 3 times daily
Atypical analgesic	Capsaicin	Topical	0.2% solution (can dilute Tabasco™ sauce) swish and expectorate 4 times daily
Supplement	Alpha-lipoic acid	Systemic	200 mg 3 times daily

Recent meta-analyses and systematic reviews of BMS therapies have cautioned that there is a paucity of high-quality research and a high risk of bias in most of the available studies. Further research is needed to develop clear guidelines and treatment recommendations for patients with BMS.[3,4,14] Based on the available evidence, practitioners should consider the individual patient and discuss appropriate possible treatment regimens.

FUTURE DIRECTIONS

Despite advances in the understanding and treatment of BMS, it remains a challenging condition for both patients and providers. Many patients visit several clinicians of varied specialty before receiving a diagnosis of BMS, with reported average delays between onset and diagnosis of anywhere from 13 to 41 months.[10,41] It is imperative that providers who encounter BMS validate their patients' symptoms and, when local and systemic causes have been ruled out, establish a diagnosis of BMS. Upon doing so, practitioners may discuss treatment options for managing symptoms.

Further research should focus on establishing treatment guidelines and best practices. In order to do so, randomized control trials conducted over longer periods with large patient populations, rigid inclusion criteria, and rigorous methods are needed. These trials should consider further investigation of treatments known to be effective in other neuropathic pain conditions as well as psychological interventions.[14]

SUMMARY

BMS is a chronic pain condition that is likely neuropathic, mediated by varied levels of dysfunction in the peripheral and central nervous system. It affects largely perimenopausal and postmenopausal women and rarely presents before the age of 30 years. A diagnosis of BMS should be made only after a thorough history, clinical examination, and indicated laboratory studies have ruled out local or systemic cause. If a causal factor is identified, treatment of the underlying condition should relieve the burning sensation. Various local, systemic, and psychological interventions have been shown to reduce BMS symptoms in both short-term and long-term intervals, although more research is needed to establish evidence-based treatment guidelines. Some patients experience at least partial remission of symptoms with or without treatment, but, for many, symptoms persist. Management should be aimed at symptom reduction and coping strategies.

DISCLOSURE

The authors have nothing to disclose.

REFERENCES

1. Grushka M, Epstein JB, Gorsky M. Burning mouth syndrome. Am Fam Physician 2002;65(4):615–20.
2. Ariyawardana A, Chmieliauskaite M, Farag AM, et al. World Workshop on Oral Medicine VII: Burning mouth syndrome: a systematic review of disease definitions and diagnostic criteria utilized in randomized clinical trials. Oral Dis 2019;25(Suppl 1): 141–56.
3. Zakrzewska J, Buchanan JA. Burning mouth syndrome. BMJ Clin Evid 2016;2016:1301.
4. Ritchie A, Kramer JM. Recent advances in the etiology and treatment of burning mouth syndrome. J Dent Res 2018;97(11):1193–9.
5. Jääskeläinen SK. Pathophysiology of primary burning mouth syndrome. Clin Neurophysiol 2012; 123(1):71–7.
6. Moghadam-Kia S, Fazel N. A diagnostic and therapeutic approach to primary burning mouth syndrome (BMS). Clin Dermatol 2017. https://doi.org/ 10.1016/j.clindermatol.2017.06.006.
7. Headache Classification Committee of the International Headache Society (IHS) the international classification of headache disorders, 3rd edition. Cephalalgia 2018;38(1):1–211.
8. Grushka M. Clinical features of burning mouth syndrome. Oral Surg Oral Med Oral Pathol 1987;63(1): 30–6.
9. Sardella A, Lodi G, Demarosi F, et al. Burning mouth syndrome: a retrospective study investigating spontaneous remission and response to treatments. Oral Dis 2006;12(2):152–5.
10. Klasser GD, Epstein JB, Villines D, et al. Burning mouth syndrome: a challenge for dental practitioners and patients. Gen Dent 2011;59(3):210–20 [quiz: 221].
11. Kolkka-Palomaa M, Jääskeläinen SK, Laine MA, et al. Pathophysiology of primary burning mouth syndrome with special focus on taste dysfunction: a review. Oral Dis 2015;21(8):937–48.
12. Patton LL, Siegel MA, Benoliel R, et al. Management of burning mouth syndrome: systematic review and management recommendations. Oral Surg Oral Med Oral Pathol Oral Radiol Endod 2007; 103(Suppl):S39.e1-13.
13. Scala A, Checchi L, Montevecchi M, et al. Update on burning mouth syndrome: overview and patient management. Crit Rev Oral Biol Med 2003;14(4): 275–91.
14. McMillan R, Forssell H, Buchanan JA, et al. Interventions for treating burning mouth syndrome. Cochrane Database Syst Rev 2016;(11):CD002779.

15. Périer JM, Boucher Y. History of burning mouth syndrome (1800-1950): A review. Oral Dis 2019;25(2): 425–38.

16. Bergdahl M, Bergdahl J. Burning mouth syndrome: prevalence and associated factors. J Oral Pathol Med 1999;28(8):350–4.

17. Kohorst JJ, Bruce AJ, Torgerson RR, et al. A population-based study of the incidence of burning mouth syndrome. Mayo Clin Proc 2014; 89(11):1545–52.

18. Lamey PJ, Lewis MA. Oral medicine in practice: burning mouth syndrome. Br Dent J 1989;167(6): 197–200.

19. Lopez-Jornet P, Molino Pagan D, Andujar Mateos P, et al. Circadian rhythms variation of pain in burning mouth syndrome. Geriatr Gerontol Int 2015;15(4): 490–5.

20. Lopez-Jornet P, Molino-Pagan D, Parra-Perez P, et al. Neuropathic pain in patients with burning mouth syndrome evaluated using painDETECT. Pain Med 2017;18(8):1528–33.

21. Gurvits GE, Tan A. Burning mouth syndrome. World J Gastroenterol 2013;19(5):665–72.

22. Lauria G, Majorana A, Borgna M, et al. Trigeminal small-fiber sensory neuropathy causes burning mouth syndrome. Pain 2005;115(3):332–7.

23. Puhakka A, Forssell H, Soinila S, et al. Peripheral nervous system involvement in primary burning mouth syndrome–results of a pilot study. Oral Dis 2016;22(4):338–44.

24. Yilmaz Z, Renton T, Yiangou Y, et al. Burning mouth syndrome as a trigeminal small fibre neuropathy: Increased heat and capsaicin receptor TRPV1 in nerve fibres correlates with pain score. J Clin Neurosci 2007;14(9):864–71.

25. Hagelberg N, Forssell H, Rinne JO, et al. Striatal dopamine D1 and D2 receptors in burning mouth syndrome. Pain 2003;101(1–2):149–54.

26. Poon R, Su N, Ching V, et al. Reduction in unstimulated salivary flow rate in burning mouth syndrome. Br Dent J 2014;217(7):E14.

27. de Moura SAB, de Sousa JMA, Lima DF, et al. Burning mouth syndrome (BMS): sialometric and sialochemical analysis and salivary protein profile. Gerodontology 2007;24(3):173–6.

28. Eliav E, Kamran B, Schaham R, et al. Evidence of chorda tympani dysfunction in patients with burning mouth syndrome. J Am Dent Assoc 2007;138(5): 628–33.

29. Nasri-Heir C, Gomes J, Heir GM, et al. The role of sensory input of the chorda tympani nerve and the number of fungiform papillae in burning mouth syndrome. Oral Surg Oral Med Oral Pathol Oral Radiol Endod 2011;112(1):65–72.

30. Bartoshuk LM, Grushka M, Duffy VB, et al. Burning mouth syndrome: damage to CN VII and pain phantoms in CN V. Chem Senses 1999;24:609.

31. Galli F, Lodi G, Sardella A, et al. Role of psychological factors in burning mouth syndrome: A systematic review and meta-analysis. Cephalalgia 2017; 37(3):265–77.

32. Adamo D, Sardella A, Varoni E, et al. The association between burning mouth syndrome and sleep disturbance: A case-control multicentre study. Oral Dis 2018;24(4):638–49.

33. López-Jornet P, Camacho-Alonso F, Andujar-Mateos P, et al. Burning mouth syndrome: an update. Med Oral Patol Oral Cir Bucal 2010;15(4): e562–8.

34. Zakrzewska JM, Buchanan JA. Burning mouth syndrome. Clin Evid 2016;2016:1301.

35. Cui Y, Xu H, Chen FM, et al. Efficacy evaluation of clonazepam for symptom remission in burning mouth syndrome: a meta-analysis. Oral Dis 2016; 22(6):503–11.

36. Heckmann SM, Kirchner E, Grushka M, et al. A double-blind study on clonazepam in patients with burning mouth syndrome. Laryngoscope 2012;122(4):813–6.

37. de Moraes M, do Amaral Bezerra BA, da Rocha Neto PC, et al. Randomized trials for the treatment of burning mouth syndrome: an evidence-based review of the literature. J Oral Pathol Med 2012;41(4): 281–7.

38. Silvestre F-J, Silvestre-Rangil J, Tamarit-Santafé C, et al. Application of a capsaicin rinse in the treatment of burning mouth syndrome. Med Oral Patol Oral Cir Bucal 2012;17(1):e1–4.

39. Saarto T, Wiffen PJ. Antidepressants for neuropathic pain. Cochrane Database Syst Rev 2007;(4): CD005454.

40. López-Jornet P, Camacho-Alonso F, Andujar-Mateos P. A prospective, randomized study on the efficacy of tongue protector in patients with burning mouth syndrome. Oral Dis 2011;17(3): 277–82.

41. Ni Riordain R, O'Dwyer S, McCreary C. Burning mouth syndrome-a diagnostic dilemma. Ir J Med Sci 2019;188(3):731–4.

Pigmented Lesions

Eugene Ko, DDS[a],*, Neeraj Panchal, DDS, MD, MA[b]

KEYWORDS

- Oral mucosa • Pigmented • Pigmentation • Melanotic • Oral medicine • Dermatology

KEY POINTS

- Introduce pigmented lesions that can present in the oral mucosa.
- Oral pigmented lesions that can overlap with cutaneous pigmented lesions.
- Underscore the differences in genetics and biological behavior of pigmented lesions that can present in both oral mucosa and cutaneous skin.
- Review the systemic diseases and diffuse presentations of pigmentation that can have oral mucosal involvement.

INTRODUCTION

There are similarities and differences in mucosal and cutaneous tissues with a range of pigmented lesions in the oral cavity correlating to diseases seen in cutaneous skin, such as melanotic macule/ephelides to cutaneous/mucosal melanomas. Ultraviolet light exposure does not seem to play a role in the development of the melanotic macule as it does with ephelis,[1] and mucosal melanoma seems to have a distinct molecular profile from that of cutaneous melanoma.[2] Cutaneous melanoacanthoma is likely a variant of seborrheic keratosis, whereas oral melanoacanthoma is not. Understanding these differences aids clinical management, because it may differ for correlate lesions. Thus, a closer look into the intricacy of oral pigmented lesions can potentially improve clinical outcomes. However, overlap in cutaneous and mucosal disease can be clinically useful. For example, the Asymmetry, Borders, Colors, Diameter, Evolving (ABCDE) checklist used for cutaneous pigmented lesions could be potentially useful to distinguish oral pigmented lesions. In addition, mucocutaneous pigmentation can occur with drug therapy, which includes biologics. In addition, a shared lexicon to describe pigmented lesions can aid in multidisciplinary care between specialties.

FOCAL PIGMENTATION
Ephelis

Definition: small pigmented spots that occur on the cutaneous skin, commonly known as freckles.

Epidemiology/pathogenesis: more commonly associated in populations with light skin and blond or red hair. Spots present during early childhood and after sun exposure, especially during summer.[3] Painful sunburns before the age of 20 years may contribute to the development of ephelides.[4]

Clinical: small, well-defined macular lesions that present commonly on the face, neck, chest, and arms that can vary in number from a few to hundreds.[5] Color varies from light brown to tan.

Investigations: several genes have been shown to be important for the formation of freckles, with MC1R shown to be a major contributor to the formation of freckles.[3,6]

[a] Department of Oral Medicine, University of Pennsylvania, School of Dental Medicine, 240 South 40th Street, Philadelphia, PA 19104, USA; [b] Department of Oral Surgery, University of Pennsylvania, School of Dental Medicine, 240 South 40th Street, Philadelphia, PA 19104, USA
* Corresponding author.
E-mail address: eugko@upenn.edu

Dermatol Clin 38 (2020) 485–494
https://doi.org/10.1016/j.det.2020.05.009

Management: treatment of ephelides is elective because they tend to fade during winter months and are removed for cosmetic reasons.[5]

Prognosis: light skin, red hair, and ephelides are indicators for an increased risk of malignant melanoma and nonmelanoma skin cancer.[3,7]

Melanotic Macule

Definition: small pigmented macule that occurs on the lips and mucosal membranes.

Epidemiology/pathogenesis: unlike the cutaneous ephelis, oral melanotic macule does not depend on sun exposure. Lesions have been reported in patients aged 1 to 98 years, with a mean of approximately 42 years. Most macules are found in female patients.[8]

Clinical: macules typically present as a solitary, well-defined lesion less than 1 cm in size. Multiple pigmented mucosal macules may indicate an underlying syndrome, such as Peutz-Jeghers.[9] Clinically, macules present as uniformly tan to brown. The lower lip vermilion border and anterior maxillary gingiva are the most common sites.[9,10]

Investigations: if a diagnosis cannot be made based on clinical presentation, a biopsy is indicated to rule out malignant mimics, such as melanoma.[11]

Management: no treatment is necessary because labial and oral melanotic macules are asymptomatic and have no malignant potential. Removal may be for cosmetic reasons or to rule out a potential mucosal melanoma, especially if lesion is on the palate, where mucosal melanomas are most prevalent.[9]

Prognosis: melanotic macules typically do not recur.[11]

MULTIFOCAL/DIFFUSE PIGMENTATION
Smoker's Melanosis

Definition: diffuse mucosal pigmentation secondary to heavy tobacco use.

Epidemiology/pathogenesis: commonly seen in female heavy smokers. Mucosal pigmentation is thought to be a protective mechanism against toxins of smoking.[8]

Clinical: most common location of pigmentation secondary to tobacco use is the labial gingiva. For pipe smokers, the most common location tends to be the buccal mucosa or the commissure of the lip along the vermilion border.[12]

Investigations: diagnosis is made through clinical correlation with the patient's smoking history.[12]

Management: the condition does not require treatment.[8]

Prognosis: smoking cessation may reduce pigmentation, typically within a 3-year period.[1,13]

Postinflammatory Pigmentation

Definition: reactive hypermelanosis of the epithelium and/or underlying connective tissue.

Epidemiology/pathogenesis: intraorally, these lesions are commonly synchronous with lichenoid inflammation (**Fig. 1**). Dark-skinned individuals are prone to developing postinflammatory pigmentation in the oral cavity.[8,11]

Clinical: characterized by pigmented macules or patches that correspond with the distribution of the original inflammation. If the pigmentation involves the epidermis, the skin appears tan or brown. Dermal hypermelanosis has a darker gray or blue-gray appearance.[14]

Investigations: a suspected case of postinflammatory pigmentation requires a search for the underlying cause, which then should be managed appropriately.[15]

Management/prognosis: most postinflammatory pigmentation tends to resolve (lighten) with time. However, topical medications may be necessary for significant improvement, such as tretinoin (retinoic acid).[15]

Melanoacanthoma

Definition: reactive melanocytic mucosal lesion that can rapidly grow and spontaneously regress.

Epidemiology/pathogenesis: oral melanoacanthoma typically occurs in African American women. The cutaneous melanoacanthoma is distinct from the oral melanoacanthoma, the former being considered a variant of seborrheic keratosis with a predilection in middle-aged white adults.[16,17]

Clinical: commonly presents as a rapidly enlarging pigmented macule on the buccal mucosa.[8,11] Other sites within the oral mucosa have

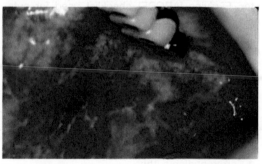

Fig. 1. Postinflammatory pigmentation and lichenoid mucositis. (*Courtesy of* Thomas P. Sollecito, DMD, FDS RCSEd, Philadelphia, PA.)

been reported, such as the gingival tissue and hard palate.[16,18]

Investigations: incisional biopsy is often indicated to rule out oral melanoma because of the rapid growth of a pigmented lesion.

Management/prognosis: melanoacanthomas typically involute following incisional biopsy or spontaneously within 2 to 6 months of diagnosis. No cases have been reported to progress to a neoplastic melanocytic process.[8,17]

Physiologic Pigmentation

Definition: racial/ethnic pigmentation of oral mucosal tissues.

Epidemiology/pathogenesis: typically observed in dark-skinned individuals.[18] The extent and intensity of pigmentation increase with age.[19]

Clinical: diffuse or localized brown macules that can involve any mucosal location, with the gingiva being the most common; when the gingiva is involved, the pigmentation is bilateral and does not extend past the mucogingival junction (**Fig. 2**).[20] When the dorsal tongue is involved, pigmentation may be limited to the fungiform papillae.[8]

Investigations: diagnosis is made on clinical examination with exclusion criteria for pigmented-related diseases.

Management/prognosis: no treatment is necessary for physiologic pigmentation.

EXOGENOUS CAUSES OF CLINICAL PIGMENTATION
Tattoos (Amalgam/Graphite/Ornamental)

Definition: pigmentation of mucosal tissues through foreign material.

Epidemiology/pathogenesis: mucosal pigmentation can occur because of deposition of exogenous foreign material either accidentally or by intention. For example, graphite from a pencil injury can lead to pigmentation.[21] In contrast, tattoo ink is used for ornamental tattooing of mucosal tissues (**Fig. 3**). However, the most common is the implantation of dental amalgam, known as an amalgam tattoo.[8,10]

Clinical: commonly presents as a blue-gray discoloration on mucosal tissues.

Investigations: radiographic images may show fragments of amalgam, which can be diagnostic.[8] Moreover, a clinical examination can be supportive of an amalgam tattoo with presence of several amalgam fillings, if radiographs do not show fragments.

Management/prognosis: no treatment indicated for pigmentation by a foreign material.

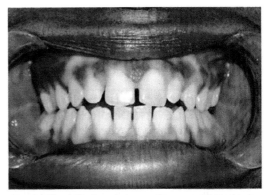

Fig. 2. Physiologic pigmentation on the gingiva. (*From* Hatch CL. Pigmented lesions of the oral cavity. Dent Clin N Am 2005;49:185-201.)

Lead Toxicity (Burton Line)

Definition: oral manifestation of lead toxicity.

Epidemiology/pathogenesis: Burton line is a sign of chronic lead intoxication that develops when lead reacts with metabolites of oral bacteria.[22] Exposure to lead is through inhalation or ingestion. Deteriorated lead-based paint in old homes are still common sources for lead exposure[23]; moreover, old homes with aging water pipes that corrode may be another source for lead. In adults, more common exposure routes are occupational or drugs that have been weighted with lead.[22,24]

Clinical: presents as a bluish line at the free gingival margin.

Investigations: blood lead levels may help to confirm lead intoxication.[22,24]

Management: treatment with chelation therapy (ie, using agents that bind to metals and remove from body through excretion) can resolve oral manifestation.

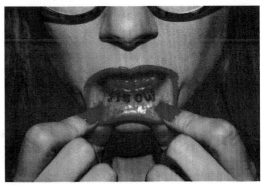

Fig. 3. Ornamental mucosal tattoo. (*Courtesy of* Eugene Ko, DDS, University of Pennsylvania, Philadelphia, PA.)

Prognosis: children are especially susceptible to lead exposure, and even low levels of exposure can cause both behavioral and cognitive deficits. Chelation therapy is unable to remediate the effect of lead on neurodevelopment.[25]

PIGMENTATIONS ASSOCIATED WITH SYSTEMIC OR GENETIC DISORDERS
Nevus (Oral Melanocytic Nevus)

Definition: uncommon, benign intraoral tumor of melanocytic lineage.

Epidemiology/pathogenesis: pigmented nevi are generally less common in the oral cavity than on the skin. Intramucosal nevi represent the most common type, followed by intraoral blue nevi. The hard palate is the most common site.[26,27]

Clinical: most melanocytic lesions measure less than 1.0 cm and are clinically flat to slightly raised.[28] All cutaneous subtypes have also been observed in the oral mucosa with the exception of the halo nevus, the pigmented spindle-cell nevus, and the deep penetrating nevus.[29]

Investigations: a biopsy is indicated to rule out malignant mimics, such as melanoma.[11]

Management: hard palate represents a common location of oral mucosal melanoma. Early mucosal melanomas can appear clinically similar to oral melanocytic nevi. Thus, biopsy is advised for pigmented oral lesions.

Prognosis: melanocytic nevi can resemble small congenital melanocytic nevi, although most congenital nevi are medium to large (1.5 cm to >20 cm). The risk of developing melanoma tends to be higher in congenital melanocytic nevi compared with acquired; however, the number of reported intraoral cases of congenital melanocytic nevi seems to be very low.[30]

Melanotic Neuroectodermal Tumor of Infancy

Definition: a rare neural crest–derived tumor occurring most often in the maxilla of infants.

Epidemiology/pathogenesis: this tumor is usually found in young children in the first year of life and with equal distribution between sexes.[31] The maxilla is the most common site.[32] However, occurrences outside of the maxilla are consistent with the wide distribution of neural crest derivatives.[33]

Clinical: commonly presents as an enlarging painless mass with a pigmented discoloration (Fig. 4).

Investigations: can be associated with increased urinary vanillylmandelic acid levels with return to normal baseline following surgical resection.[32] However, increased levels of vanillylmandelic acid can be found in other tumors with neural crest origin, such as neuroblastomas. In most patients, presurgical values of vanillylmandelic acid were normal.[34] There has been a lack of molecular links to other pediatric neural crest tumors.[35]

Management: surgical removal is the mainstay of treatment; however, in infants, wide excision may be associated with significant mutilation. Thus, there is debate whether wide surgical excision is necessary in all cases because some tumor islets have been reported to have regressed after incomplete excision.[34]

Prognosis: infants who were diagnosed within the first 2 months of birth had a shorter disease-free survival time, and all recurrences occurred within 6 months of treatment. In contrast, children diagnosed after 4.5 months of age had a minimal risk of recurrence.[36] Older patients likely underwent more radical surgery, which was associated with a lower recurrence rate, in contrast with younger patients.[34]

Oral Mucosal Melanoma

Definition: malignant neoplasm of melanocytes in the oral mucosa.

Epidemiology: oral mucosal melanoma is uncommon because less than 1% present as primary lesions in the oral cavity. Mucosal melanomas do not share the environmental risk factor (ie, ultraviolet radiation) that is seen in cutaneous and ocular melanomas.[37] Moreover, the cause and pathogenesis are poorly understood and no intraoral risk factor has been recognized to date.[38] Rates of mucosal melanoma seem to be higher among white people than among black people.[37]

Clinical: clinically, most oral mucosal melanomas are diagnosed as pigmented nodular lesions (Fig. 5). A classification of the 5 varied presentations of oral mucosal melanoma has been proposed: (1) pigmented nodular, (2) nonpigmented nodular, (3) pigmented macular, (4) pigmented mixed, and (5) nonpigmented mixed.[39] The most common sites are the hard palate and gingiva.[38]

Investigations: most oral melanomas arise de novo from apparently normal mucosa, and a definite precursor lesion has not yet been identified.[38] The molecular profile is distinct from cutaneous melanoma with higher rates of KIT mutations, followed by NRAS mutations, and rare BRAF mutations.[40]

Management: currently, radical resection of the primary tumor is the treatment of choice. Unlike cutaneous melanoma, guidelines are not available for the optimal width of tumor-free margins. Moreover, controversy remains on the

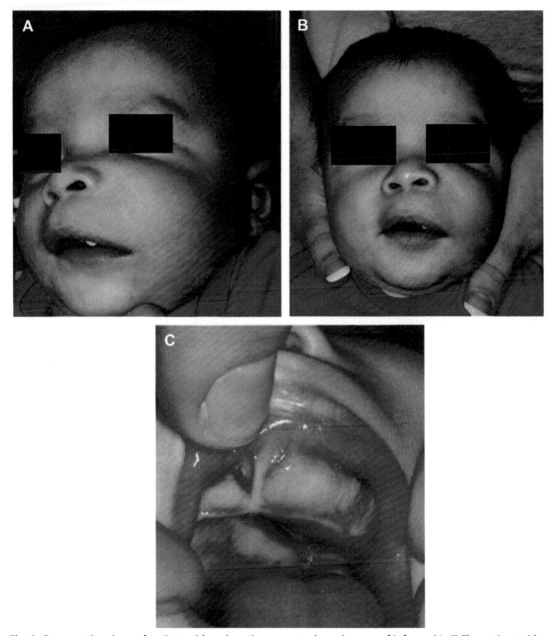

Fig. 4. Preoperative views of patient with melanotic neuroectodermal tumor of infancy. (*A, B*) The patient with a left maxillary mass at presentation to the clinic. (*C*) Intraoral view of tumor extruding from the hard palate and alveolar process. (*From* Rachidi S, Sood AJ, Patel KG et al. J Oral Maxillofac Surg 2015;73:1946-1956; with permission.)

issue of prophylactic neck dissection because there is no evidence yet that elective nodal dissection improves survival. However, risk of cervical lymph node involvement is higher in oral mucosal melanoma than in other mucosal melanomas of the head and neck, which supports elective neck dissection.[41,42] Surgery may be combined with radiotherapy, chemotherapy, or immunotherapy, although the effectiveness of such therapies, both as primary therapy and in association with the surgical treatment, is largely unknown.[41]

Prognosis: oral mucosal melanoma presents with frequent metastasis and a 5-year survival ranging from 15% to 40%.[38] Clinical stage (extent of tumor, regional lymph nodes, and distant metastasis) at presentation is probably the most important factor in determining outcome.[41,42]

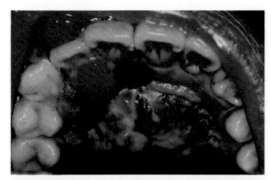

Fig. 5. Mucosal melanoma of the hard palate. (*From* Malinoski H, Reddy R, Cohen DM et al. J Oral Maxillofac Surg 2019;77:1832-1936; with permission.)

Addison Disease

Definition: Addison disease (primary adrenal insufficiency, hypocortisolism) is an endocrine condition in which adrenal dysfunction results in decreased endogenous corticosteroid levels.

Epidemiology/pathogenesis: the adrenal gland has a feedback loop with the pituitary gland. The anterior pituitary gland synthesizes adrenocorticotropic hormone (ACTH) with decreased level of corticosteroids. The ACTH acts on the adrenal gland to stimulate production of corticosteroids. Via the feedback loop, the corticosteroid increase from the adrenal gland decreases production of ACTH from the anterior pituitary gland. When there is dysfunction of the adrenal gland, there is persistent ACTH production from the anterior pituitary gland. The alpha-melanocyte–stimulating hormone (α-MSH) gene is an alternatively spliced gene originating from the same gene as ACTH. An increase in ACTH production concomitantly results in an increase in α-MSH. α-MSH stimulates melanocytes to produce melanin, resulting in diffuse mucocutaneous pigmentation.[43] Addison disease has no predilection for age, sex, or ethnicity; however, it typically presents in middle-aged adults. The frequency of the disease is estimated at 0.6 per 100,000 person-years. The prevalence is estimated at 14 per 100,000 persons.[44]

Clinical: acute primary adrenal insufficiency presents with orthostatic hypotension, agitation, confusion, circulatory collapse, abdominal pain, and fever. Typical causes of acute primary adrenal insufficiency include hemorrhage, metastasis, and acute infection. In contrast, chronic primary adrenal insufficiency presents as malaise, fatigue, anorexia, weight loss, joint and back pain, and darkening of the skin. The darkening of the skin can be homogeneous or blotchy, but can especially occur in the sun-exposed areas.

Mucocutaneous pigmentation can be one of the earliest clinical manifestations. The skin can have a bronze appearance, especially in fair-skinned individuals.[43] In the oral cavity, there can be patchy melanosis of multiple mucosal surfaces, including the tongue, gingiva, buccal mucosa, and hard palate. The macules can present as blue-black or brown and can have a spotty or streaked patterned.[43]

Investigations: systemic diagnosis can initially be suspected, with routine laboratory testing showing hypoglycemia, hyponatremia, hyperkalemia, eosinophilia, and lymphocytosis and metabolic acidosis. Systemic diagnosis can be confirmed with an ACTH stimulation test. The diagnosis of the pigmented lesion requires a clinicopathologic correlation.[43,45]

Management/prognosis: lifelong steroid replacement therapy typically results in a decrease in cutaneous pigmentation; however, oral pigmentation may still persist indefinitely.[46]

Cushing Disease

Definition: Cushing disease is characterized by increased secretion of ACTH, thus also α-MSH, from the anterior pituitary, often as a result of a pituitary adenoma.

Epidemiology/pathogenesis: the increased ACTH can also present from overproduction of corticotropin-releasing hormone from the hypothalamus. It is important to differentiate Cushing syndrome from prolonged exposure to high concentrations of endogenous or exogenous corticosteroids. Cushing syndrome can be as a result of adrenal disorder, iatrogenic prolonged steroid exposure, or Cushing disease. Oral pigmentation is only present in Cushing syndrome if it is a result of Cushing disease.[47] Cushing disease is extremely rare in children and typically presents in the third and fourth decades of life. The annual incidence of benign adrenal adenoma causing Cushing disease is 0.6 per million.[48]

Clinical: Cushing disease presents systemically with weight gain, hypertension, diabetes mellitus, osteoporosis, muscle atrophy, dyslipidemia kidney stones, and moon facies. Similar to Addison disease, there can be patchy melanosis of multiple mucosal surfaces or spotty or streaked macules.

Investigations: diagnosis of Cushing disease requires initial diagnosis of Cushing syndrome via dexamethasone suppression testing or cortisol levels, and then ACTH level and brain imaging confirmation to indicate Cushing disease.[49]

Management/prognosis: the oral manifestations of Cushing disease subside after the surgical management of the pituitary disorder.

Peutz-Jeghers Syndrome

Definition: Peutz-Jeghers syndrome is an autosomal dominant disorder of germline mutations in the STK11/LKB1 tumor suppressor gene resulting in intestinal hamartomatous polyposis and increased susceptibility to multiple neoplasms.[50]

Epidemiology/pathogenesis: it has an estimated prevalence of approximately 1 in 8000 to 200,000 births. The average age of first diagnosis is 23 years; however, diagnosis can be recognized in childhood. Men and women are equally affected.[50]

Clinical: an early clinical manifestation of the syndrome is labial, perioral, and acral macular pigmentation that mimics dark freckling. Pigmentation inside the mouth is uncommon. The pattern of lip and perioral pigmentation is similar to Laugier-Hunziker pigmentation (discussed later).[51] Whenever this pattern is identified, further exploration of family history and genetic testing may be needed. Rectal bleeding or other gastrointestinal complaints warrant referral to a gastroenterologist. Other initial presentations may include bowel obstruction with intussusception.[52]

Management/prognosis: patients with Peutz-Jeghers syndrome require cancer surveillance along with continual observation with a gastroenterologist. The pigmentation will persist, but can be improved with laser therapy.[53]

Laugier-Hunziker Pigmentation

Definition: Laugier-Hunziker pigmentation is multifocal pigmentation of the labial and buccal mucosae with no other potential systemic sources of pigmentation. It is a diagnosis of exclusion.[51]

Epidemiology/pathogenesis: the idiopathic pigmentation has no sex or racial predilection and is typically identified in adulthood. The pigmentation is caused by an accumulation of melanin in the basal layer keratinocytes and an increase in the number of melanophages in the submucosa and/or papillary dermis.[54]

Clinical: patients present with multiple, small, discrete, irregular, darkly pigmented macules. Other mucosal surfaces within the mouth, esophagus, genitalia, and conjunctiva may also show the pigmentation. Melanotic streaks of the nails can be seen and, in rare cases, pigmentation changes of the acral skin surfaces.

Management/prognosis: all systemic causes of the pigmentation must initially be ruled out. Once other diagnoses have been ruled out, laser therapy may be beneficial to improve cosmetics.[51]

Neurofibromatosis

Definition: neurofibromatosis (NF) is an autosomal dominant genetic disorder characterized by multiple cutaneous lesions and tumors of the nervous system with 2 specific subtypes, NF-1 and NF-2.[55]

Epidemiology/pathogenesis: NF-1 affects approximately 1 in 3500 individuals. Half of affected patients have a positive family history and the other half are from a spontaneous mutation of the NF-1 gene on chromosome 17.[55]

Clinical: NF-1 presents with light brown macules of approximately 10 to 40 mm with an ovoid shape. The presence of 6 macules is a strong diagnosis criterion. Other common findings include axillary and inguinal freckling, neurofibromas of peripheral nerves, and Lisch nodules (pigmented hamartomas of the iris). Patients may have congenital musculoskeletal disorders at birth. Intraorally patients have unilateral fibrous gingiva and symmetric melanin pigmentation of the gingiva. There can be impacted teeth, supernumerary teeth, missing teeth, and overgrowth of the alveolar process.[56]

Management/prognosis: NF-1 has no cure but is continually followed by a team of specialists. Laser therapy may aid in cosmesis of the gingival pigmentation.

Human Immunodeficiency Virus Kaposi Sarcoma

Definition: Oral Kaposi sarcoma (KS) is a multifocal vascular malignancy seen in patients with a diagnosis of acquired immunodeficiency syndrome (AIDS) caused by human herpesvirus 8. The mouth may be affected in all KS variants, but is most often seen with AIDS.

Epidemiology/pathogenesis: the incidence in men and women is equal. As CD-4 T-cell counts decrease, the incidence of KS increases. The use of highly active antiretroviral therapy (HAART) has dramatically decreased the incidence of KS.[57] Early-stage KS is characterized by many small abnormal vessels dissecting tissue. More advanced KS histology shows a proliferation of spindle-shaped cells surrounding poorly formed vascular spaces or slits with extravasated red blood cells. Well-developed KS shows fascicles of spindle-shaped tumor cells. Immunohistochemistry shows staining for endothelial markers such as factor VIII–related antigen; CD31 and CD34; and lymphatic-specific markers such as D2-40, LYVE-1, VEGF4-3, and Prox-1. The most diagnostic marker is identification of human herpesvirus 8 with commercially available antibody LNA-1.[57,58]

Clinical: KS commonly affects the hard palate, gingiva, and tongue. Early lesions are flat or slightly elevated brown to purple lesions that are often bilateral. Advanced lesions are dark red to purple plaques or nodules that may show ulceration, bleeding, and necrosis. The lesions may be unifocal or multifocal and can be indolent or rapidly progressive.[59]

Management/prognosis: human immunodeficiency virus–associated KS is managed with HAART and systemic chemotherapy. In some situations, surgical excision, intralesional chemotherapy, intralesional sclerosing agents, photodynamic therapy, and cryosurgery may be necessary to manage the lesions locally.[57,60]

Hemochromatosis

Definition: hemochromatosis (bronze diabetes) is an inherited autosomal recessive disorder caused by a mutation in the HFE gene with increase iron absorption resulting in diabetes, heart failure, and cirrhosis.[61]

Epidemiology/pathogenesis: hemochromatosis is one of the most common heritable genetic conditions in people of northern European descent, with a prevalence of 1 in 200.[62]

Clinical: the hyperpigmentation of the skin associated with hemochromatosis can be brown, bronze, or slate gray. Twenty-five percent of patients have an intraoral bluish-gray pigmentation of the hard palate and possibly the gingiva.[61] The pigmentation is likely caused by melanin deposition.

Investigations: diagnostic studies showing serum ferritin levels greater than 200 μg/L in premenopausal women and 300 μg/L in men. A fasting transferrin saturation (serum iron/total iron binding capacity) greater than 45% to 50% is diagnostic.[61,63,64]

Management/prognosis: hemochromatosis is managed generally with phlebotomy and, when this is not possible, chelation therapy with desferrioxamine mesylate. Desferrioxamine mesylate is an iron chelating agent. Vitamin C administration can result in further iron excretion.[61]

SUMMARY

Dermatologists frequently encounter oral pigmented lesions within their practices. This article serves as a resource for clinicians and, if ambiguity or uncertainty exists, then referral to an oral health care provider with experience in the management of pigmented lesions should be considered.

DISCLOSURE

The authors have nothing to disclose.

REFERENCES

1. Stoopler ET, Alawi F. Pigmented lesions of the oral mucosa. In: Farah C, Balasubramaniam R, McCullough M, editors. Contemporary oral medicine. Cham (Switzerland): Springer; 2019. p. 1178–9.
2. Williams MD. Update from the 4th edition of the World Health Organization classification of head and neck tumors: mucosal melanomas. Head Neck Pathol 2017;11:110–7.
3. Bastiaens M, ter Huurne J, Gruis N, et al. The melanocortin-1-receptor gene is the major freckle gene. Hum Mol Genet 2001;10:1701–8.
4. Bastiaens M, Hoefnagel J, Westendorp R, et al. Solar lentigines are strongly related to sun exposure in contrast to ephelides. Pigment Cell Res 2004;17:225–9.
5. Plensdorf S, Martinez J. Common pigmentation disorders. Am Fam Physician 2009;79:109–16.
6. Praetorius C, Sturm RA, Steingrimsson E. Sun-induced freckling: ephelides and solar lentigines. Pigment Cell Melanoma Res 2014;27:339–50.
7. Bliss JM, Ford D, Swerdlow AJ, et al. Risk of cutaneous melanoma associated with pigmentation characteristics and freckling: systematic overview of 10 case-control studies. Int J Cancer 1995;62:367–76.
8. Rosebush MS, Briody AN, Cordell KG. Black and brown: non-neoplastic pigmentation of the oral mucosa. Head Neck Pathol 2019;13:47–55.
9. Buchner A, Merrell PW, Carpenter WM. Relative frequency of solitary melanocytic lesions of the oral mucosa. J Oral Pathol Med 2004;33:550–7.
10. Tavares TS, Meirelles DP, de Aguiar MCF, et al. Pigmented lesions of the oral mucosa: a cross sectional study of 458 histopathological specimens. Oral Dis 2018;24:1484–91.
11. Alawi F. Pigmented lesions of the oral cavity: an update. Dent Clin North Am 2013;57:699–710.
12. Muller S. Melanin-associated pigmented lesions of the oral mucosa: presentation, differential diagnosis, and treatment. Dermatol Ther 2010;23:220–9.
13. Hedin CA, Pindborg JJ, Axell T. Disappearance of smoker's melanosis after reducing smoking. J Oral Pathol Med 1993;22:228–30.
14. Callender VD, St Surin-Lord S, Davis EC, et al. Post-inflammatory hyperpigmentation. Am J Clin Dermatol 2011;12:87–99.
15. Taylor S, Grimes P, Lim J, et al. Postinflammatory hyperpigmentation. J Cutan Med Surg 2009;13:183–91.
16. Peters SM, Mandel L, Perrino MA. Oral melanoacanthoma of the palate: an unusual presentation of an uncommon entity. JAAD Case Rep 2018;4:138–9.
17. Fornatora ML, Reich RF, Haber S, et al. Oral melanoacanthoma. Am J Dermatopathol 2003;25:12–5.

18. Stoopler ET, Ojeda D, Alawi F. Asymptomatic pigmented lesions of the gingiva. JAMA Derm 2017; 153:1045–6.

19. Feller L, Masilana A, Khammissa RAG, et al. Melanin: the biophysiology of oral melanocytes and physiological oral pigmentation. Head Face Med 2014;10:1–7.

20. Masilana A, Khammissa RAG, Lemmer J, et al. Physiological oral melanin pigmentation in a South African sample: a clinical study. J Investig Clin Dent 2017;8:1–6.

21. Yeta N, Yeta EN, Önder C, et al. Graphite tattoo on the gingiva: a case report. Clin Adv Periodontics 2016;6:140–5.

22. Helmich F, Lock G. Burton's line from chronic lead intoxication. N Engl J Med 2018;379:e35.

23. Pearce JMS. Burton's line in lead poisoning. Eur Neurol 2007;57:118–9.

24. Chawla MPS, Sundriyal D. Burton's line. N Engl J Med 2012;367:937.

25. Neal AP, Guilarte TR. Mechanisms of lead and manganese neurotoxicity. Toxicol Res 2013;2:99–114.

26. Buchner A, Hansen LS. Pigmented nevi of the oral mucosa: a clinicopathologic study of 32 new cases and review of 75 cases from the literature. Part II. Analysis of 107 cases. Oral Surg Oral Med Oral Pathol 1980;49:55–62.

27. Fistarol SK, Itin PH. Plaque-type blue nevus of the oral cavity. Dermatology 2005;211:224–33.

28. Ferreira L, Jham B, Assi R, et al. Oral melanocytic nevi: a clinicopathologic study of 100 cases. Oral Surg Oral Med Oral Pathol Oral Radiol 2015;120: 358–67.

29. Amérigo-Góngora M, Machuca-Portillo G, Torres-Lagares D, et al. Clinicopathological and immunohistochemical analysis of oral melanocytic nevi and review of the literature. J Stomatol Oral Maxillofac Surg 2017;118:151–5.

30. Torres KG, Carle L, Royer M. Nevus spilus (speckled lentiginous nevus) in the oral cavity: report of a case and review of the literature. Am J Dermatopathol 2017;39:e8–12.

31. Kruse-Losler B, Gaertner C, Burger H, et al. Melanotic neuroectodermal tumor of infancy: systematic review of the literature and presentation of a case. Oral Surg Oral Med Oral Pathol Oral Radiol Endod 2006;102:204–16.

32. Soles BS, Wilson A, Lucas D, et al. Melanotic neuroectodermal tumor of infancy. Arch Pathol Lab Med 2018;142:1358–63.

33. Nikai H, Ijuhin N, Yamasaki A, et al. Ultrastructural evidence for neural crest origin of the melanotic neuroectodermal tumor of infancy. J Oral Path 1977;6: 221–32.

34. Chrcanovic BR, Gomez RS. Melanotic tumor of infancy of the jaw: an analysis of diagnostic features and treatment. Int J Oral Maxillofac Surg 2019;48:1–8.

35. Khoddami M, Squire J, Zielenska M, et al. Melanotic neuroectodermal tumor of infancy: a molecular genetic study. Pediatr Dev Pathol 1998;1:295–9.

36. Rachidi S, Sood AJ, Patel KG, et al. Melanotic neuroectodermal tumor of infancy: a systematic review. J Oral Maxillofac Surg 2015;73:1946–56.

37. McLaughlin CC, Wu XC, Jemal A, et al. Incidence of noncutaneous melanomas in the U.S. Cancer 2005; 103:1000–7.

38. Sortino-Rachou AM, de Carmargo Cancela M, Voti L, et al. Primary oral melanoma: population based-incidence. Oral Oncol 2009;45:254–8.

39. Tanaka N, Mimura M, Kimijima Y, et al. Clinical investigation of amelanotic malignant melanoma in the oral region. J Oral Maxillofac Surg 2004;62:933–7.

40. El-Naggar AK, Chan JKC, Grandis JR, et al. World Health Organization classification of head and neck tumors. 4th edition. Lyon (France): IARC; 2017.

41. Meleti M, Leemans CR, Mooi WJ. Oral malignant melanoma: a review of the literature. Oral Oncol 2007;43:116–21.

42. Chatzistefanou I, Kolokythas A, Vahtsevanos K, et al. Primary mucosal melanoma of the oral cavity: current therapy and future direction. Oral Surg Oral Med Oral Pathol Oral Radiol 2016;122:17–27.

43. Shah SS, Oh CH, Coffin SE, et al. Addisonian pigmentation of the oral mucosa. Cutis 2005;76(2): 97–9.

44. Cooper GS, Stroehla BC. The epidemiology of autoimmune diseases. Autoimmun Rev 2003;2(3): 119–25.

45. Nieman LK, Chanco Turner ML. Addison's disease. Clin Dermatol 2006;24(4):276–80.

46. Dummett CO. Systemic significance of oral pigmentation and discoloration. Postgrad Med 1971;49(1): 78–82.

47. Newell-Price J, Bertagna X, Grossman AB, et al. Cushing's syndrome. Lancet 2006;367(9522): 1605–17.

48. Lindholm J, Juul S, Jorgensen JOL, et al. Incidence and late prognosis of Cushing's syndrome: a population-based study. J Clin Endocrinol Metab 2001; 86:117–23.

49. Shah KR, Boland CR, Patel M, et al. Cutaneous manifestations of gastrointestinal disease: part I. J Am Acad Dermatol 2013;68(2):189.e1-21 [quiz: 210].

50. Lindor NM, Greene MH. The concise handbook of family cancer syndromes. Mayo Familial Cancer Program. J Natl Cancer Inst 1998;90(14): 1039–71.

51. Lampe AK, Hampton PJ, Woodford-Richens K, et al. Laugier-Hunziker syndrome: an important differential diagnosis for Peutz-Jeghers syndrome. J Med Genet 2003;40(6):e77.

52. Higham P, Alawi F, Stoopler ET. Medical management update: Peutz Jeghers syndrome. Oral Surg

Oral Med Oral Pathol Oral Radiol Endod 2010;
109(1):5–11.

53. DePadova-Elder SM, Milgraum SS. Q-switched ruby
laser treatment of labial lentigines in Peutz-Jeghers
syndrome. J Dermatol Surg Oncol 1994;20(12):
830–2.

54. Mignogna MD, Lo Muzio L, Ruoppo E, et al. Oral
manifestations of idiopathic lenticular mucocutaneous pigmentation (Laugier-Hunziker syndrome):
a clinical, histopathological and ultrastructural review of 12 cases. Oral Dis 1999;5(1):80–6.

55. Gerber PA, Antal AS, Neumann NJ, et al. Neurofibromatosis. Eur J Med Res 2009;14(3):102–5.

56. Javed F, Ramalingam S, Ahmed HB, et al. Oral manifestations in patients with neurofibromatosis type-1:
a comprehensive literature review. Crit Rev Oncol
Hematol 2014;91(2):123–9.

57. Pantanowitz L, Khammissa RAG, Lemmer J, et al.
Oral HIV-associated Kaposi sarcoma. J Oral Pathol
Med 2013;42(3):201–7.

58. Flaitz CM, Jin YT, Hicks MJ, et al. Kaposi's sarcoma-
associated herpesvirus-like DNA sequences (KSHV/
HHV-8) in oral AIDS-Kaposi's sarcoma: a PCR and

clinicopathologic study. Oral Surg Oral Med Oral
Pathol Oral Radiol Endod 1997;83(2):259–64.

59. Nichols CM, Flaitz CM, Hicks MJ. Treating Kaposi's
lesions in the HIV-infected patient. J Am Dent Assoc
1993;124(11):78–84.

60. Tappero JW, Berger TG, Kaplan LD, et al. Cryotherapy for cutaneous Kaposi's sarcoma (KS) associated with acquired immune deficiency syndrome
(AIDS): a phase II trial. J Acquir Immune Defic Syndr
1991;4(9):839–46.

61. Bacon BR, Adams PC, Kowdley KV, et al. American
Association for the Study of Liver Diseases. Diagnosis and management of hemochromatosis: 2011
practice guideline by the American Association for
the Study of Liver Diseases. Hepatology 2011;
54(1):328–43.

62. EASL clinical practice guidelines for HFE hemochromatosis. Available at: https://www.ncbi.nlm.nih.
gov/pubmed/20471131. Accessed December 9,
2019.

63. Perdrup A, Poulsen H. Hemochromatosis and viti-
ligo. Arch Dermatol 1964;90:34–7.

64. Lenane P, Powell FC. Oral pigmentation. J Eur Acad
Dermatol Venereol 2000;14(6):448–65.

Oral Manifestations of Systemic Diseases

Joel J. Napeñas, DDS, FDSRCS(Ed)[a],*, Michael T. Brennan, DDS, MHS, FDSRCS(Ed)[a],
Sharon Elad, DMD, MSc[b]

KEYWORDS

- Systemic • Oral ulcers • Xerostomia • Sjogren's syndrome • Cancer

KEY POINTS

- Gastrointestinal disorders may manifest in the oral cavity as oral ulcerations, subjective or objective changes in salivary function, sensory changes, and direct impact on the dentition.
- Hematologic disorders may manifest as infiltration-type or compression-type lesions that affect adjacent organs, or consequences of the damage to specific blood lineages.
- Endocrine conditions that may impact the orofacial region include those that affect the adrenal glands, thyroid glands, parathyroid glands, diabetes, and disorders associated with growth hormones.
- Nutritional deficiencies manifest in the oral cavity as oral ulcerations, changes in soft tissue architecture or integrity, sensory changes, or increased risk of infectious tendencies.
- Infectious conditions of viral, fungal and bacterial origin in the orofacial region are generally more prevalent in immunocompromised or immunosuppressed individuals.

INTRODUCTION

Systemic conditions presenting in the orofacial region may be the initial sign of an acute or chronic systemic condition that was not previously diagnosed. Pathologic processes in the mouth, jaws, and contiguous structures could have a direct or indirect impact on the patient's overall systemic condition. In addition, these processes may directly affect the function of the orofacial structures and patients' dentition and periodontium. Medical management of systemic conditions may have implications on the orofacial region. This article reviews selected systemic conditions that present or impact the oral cavity and orofacial region.

GASTROINTESTINAL DISORDERS

As the upper anatomic region of the gastrointestinal track, the oral cavity may exhibit manifestations of systemic gastrointestinal disorders, such as those seen in inflammatory bowel disease (covered in another chapter). Such gastrointestinal disturbances can have an impact on the oral mucosal tissues.

Gastroesophageal Reflux Disease

Oral complaints in patients with gastroesophageal reflux disease include periodic sialorrhea (hypersalivation), xerostomia (subjective feeling of dry mouth), burning sensation with redness, tongue sensitivity, halitosis (bad breath), globus sensation, dysgeusia (altered taste), odynophagia and dental thermal sensitivity. Oral mucosal findings include erythema and ulcerations, typically on the palate and uvula.[1] Gingivitis, periodontitis, and dental erosion leading to thermal sensitivity and/or pulpitis of the teeth are sequelae of gastroesophageal reflux disease

[a] Department of Oral Medicine, Atrium Health's Carolinas Medical Center, PO Box 32861, Charlotte, NC 28232, USA; [b] Division of Oral Medicine, Hospital Dentistry, Eastman Institute for Oral Health, University of Rochester Medical Center, 625 Elmwood Avenue, Rochester, NY 14620, USA
* Corresponding author.
E-mail address: joel.napenas@atriumhealth.org

Dermatol Clin 38 (2020) 495–505
https://doi.org/10.1016/j.det.2020.05.010

affecting the dentition and periodontium. Dental erosion occurs owing to loss of tooth substance from exposure to gastric acid. This process can lead to hypersensitivity, functional impairment, and even tooth fracture. In gastroesophageal reflux disease, erosion commonly occurs on the occlusal surfaces of the posterior mandibular teeth and the palatal surfaces of the maxillary anterior teeth (**Fig. 1**).

Liver Disease

Oral manifestations of cirrhotic liver disease include jaundice or prolonged bleeding owing to platelet sequestration or coagulopathy. Patients with jaundice have a diffuse, uniform, yellow discoloration of all mucosal surfaces, most prominent on the lingual frenum and soft palate (**Fig. 2**). Owing to thrombocytopenia or coagulopathies, oral manifestations may include petechiae, hemorrhage, and gingival bleeding, or blood originating from esophageal varices (see Bleeding Disorders, elsewhere in this article).

Sialadenosis, an asymptomatic bilateral enlargement of the parotid glands not related to inflammatory or neoplastic processes, has been most often associated with alcoholic liver disease and alcoholic cirrhosis,[2] however, it has also been associated with nonalcoholic cirrhosis.[3] This finding may be attributed to malnutrition and metabolic abnormalities that lead to autonomic neuropathy.

Lichen planus (LP) has been associated with hepatitis C virus (HCV) infection, with patients with LP reported to have a 5 times higher risk for HCV seropositivity. The general prevalence of liver disease (not confined to HCV) in patients with LP has ranged from 0.1% to 35.0%, with the erosive variant of LP being predominant.[4] Although the mechanism is not clear, it is suggested that it is

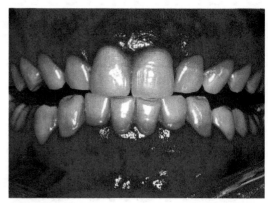

Fig. 2. Jaundice as seen in the oral mucosa and gingiva in a patient with end-stage liver disease.

due to cell-mediated cytotoxicity, in which HCV may induce cytokine and lymphokine activity.[5]

HEMATOLOGIC DISEASES
Anemia

In the mouth, anemia may manifest as pallor of the oral mucosa or loss of tongue papillation. The patient may describe tongue soreness, burning, or tingling associated with loss of papillation. Anemia may also trigger the development of aphthous ulcerations.[6] These lesions have a round/elliptical shape, with a central fibrinous pseudomembrane and an erythematous border. Minor aphthous ulcers have a diameter up to 10 mm (**Fig. 3**), whereas in major aphthous ulcers, lesions are larger and have a less-defined shape. The least common type of aphthous ulcer is herpetiform,

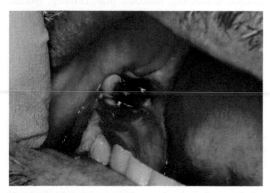

Fig. 1. Acid erosion on the occlusal surfaces of the mandibular posterior teeth in a patient with gastroesophageal reflux disease.

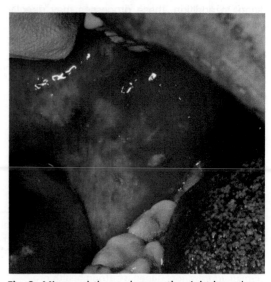

Fig. 3. Minor aphthous ulcer on the right buccal mucosa, that is, less than 10 mm.

where the ulcers are the size of a pin head, occur in clusters, but are not associated with herpes simplex virus (HSV) infection (**Fig. 4**).

Iron deficiency anemia (also covered elsewhere in this article) has several oral manifestations, including taste change (dysgeusia), taste loss (ageusia), and angular cheilitis.[7] In patients with comorbidities and polypharmacy, which can also confer similar symptoms, it may be challenging to diagnose and treat.

In thalassemia, an accumulation of excess globin chains leads to erythrocytes that undergo cell lysis, leading to a microcytic, hypochromic anemia. The bone marrow spaces in the maxillofacial complex are larger, with reduced trabeculation, and hair-on-end appearance on skull radiographs. Consequently, the bone marrow hyperplasia occurs at the expense of the anatomic sinuses, which enlarges the alveolar processes, thins the cortical bone, shrinks the maxillary sinus, and leads to bimaxillary protrusion and a spaced dentition.[8] Owing to repeated multiple blood transfusions and iron deposits in the tissues, the color may seem to be light brown or bronze and salivary gland function may be compromised, leading to hyposalivation.[9]

Bleeding Disorders

Bleeding disorders can be classified as platelet disorders, coagulopathies, and disorders of the blood vessel wall. Oral bleeding may be inadvertently triggered by normal oral function and may require pharmacologic or surgical intervention to control it. Sites most prone to trauma are adjacent to the teeth on the occlusal plane, such as the buccal mucosa and labial mucosa. The oral manifestations include petechiae (**Fig. 5**) on mucosal surfaces, submucosal bleeding or fresh bleeding into the oral cavity (eg, bloody-pinkish saliva, gingival oozing, or active bleeding from traumatized soft tissues), or the deposit of dried or clotted blood (eg, crusting on the lips, soft liver clots in the gingival or oral surfaces). Purpura most commonly develops in the soft palate, and it is possible that they are caused by friction and suction during swallowing. Perioral or submandibular hematomas may develop in response to palpation or light pressure. Bleeding into the temporomandibular joint and associated disrupted growth causing limited oral function was previously of concern in patients with hemophilia. However, with advances in the treatment for hemophilia, this complication is now extremely rare.[10]

Impaired clot degradation may occur in fibrinolytic disorders, manifesting as gingival bleeding with swelling and ulceration,[11] or a thin film of fibrin may be present along the gingivae.[12]

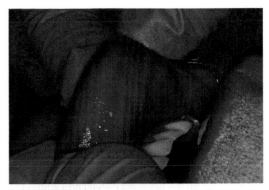

Fig. 4. Herpetiform ulcers seen in a patient in the absence of viral etiology.

Hematologic Malignancies

The white blood count may be quantitative or qualitative. Furthermore, myeloablative cancer treatment may affect white blood cell count and function. The red blood cell and platelet lineages may also be affected in hematologic malignancies.

Fungal, viral, and bacterial infections in the oral tissues are common in immunosuppressed patients (see section on Infectious Diseases) A common bacterial infection involving the gingival area surrounding a partially erupted tooth and the edentulous ridge is termed pericoronitis. Deep periodontal pockets around these teeth are common in this location and infection owing to bacterial accumulation in these pockets often occurs in immunocompromised patients.

Gingival enlargement may develop owing to leukemic infiltrate. Accumulation of leukemic cells in a form of a solid mass is termed granulocytic sarcoma or chloroma. This mass may disturb chewing and become ulcerated after dental

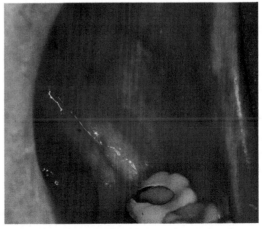

Fig. 5. Petechiae on the left buccal mucosa of a patient with thrombocytopenia owing to liver disease.

trauma. The abnormal anatomy may enable plaque accumulation. In thrombocytopenic patients, the bulky gingivae tend to bleed or show minor hematomas.

Microscopic infiltration of the leukemic cells around the nerves or compression effects of the leukemic infiltrate next to the nerves innervating the orofacial tissues may result in neuropathy. This neuropathy manifests as paresthesia, anesthesia, or burning pain.

In multiple myeloma and lymphoma, there may be a mass effect owing to compression of the malignant mass on the adjacent nerves and leading to loss of sensory or motor function. Superficial plasmacytomas or lymphomas may present as painless, raised masses. When the lesion is central to bone on imaging, a radiolucent lesion will be noted. In multiple-myeloma, the bony lesions have a well-defined border (punched-out lesions), whereas in lymphoma, the radiologic border tends to be poorly defined. Most oral lymphomas develop in the tonsils or the parotid gland,[13] but can also occur within the jawbones. In the endemic type of Burkitt lymphoma, also known as African type, maxillary involvement is common, and expansion of the body of the mandible may also occur.[14]

Langerhans cell histiocytosis is characterized by the proliferation of immature dendritic cells, the Langerhans cell histiocytes. It is rare, with oral manifestations predominantly affecting patients less than 40 years of age.[15] Nonspecific ulcerated lesions may be the only manifestation of Langerhans cell histiocytosis; therefore, a final confirmatory diagnosis is to be performed based on histopathology. Another oral manifestation of Langerhans cell histiocytosis is alveolar bone destruction. These radiolucent lesions are typically in a shape of a tub surrounding the roots of the molars, causing a floating appearance to the affected teeth. Clinically, this condition may resemble a localized gingival recession or periodontal disease. The abnormal gingival anatomy tends to trap dental plaque and secondary gingivitis complicates the presentation, accompanied by tooth mobility.

ENDOCRINE DISEASES

Because the field of endocrinology encompasses numerous glands and hormones with a plethora of functions, the orofacial manifestations of endocrine diseases are numerous and varied.

Hypothalamus–Pituitary Gland

The hypothalamus controls pituitary gland function and secretion of several hormones, each with its own oral manifestations when dysregulated. There may also be primary dysfunction in the target organs (eg, adrenal, thyroid), with oral manifestations related to these specific organs as discussed elsewhere in this article.

Adrenal Gland

Hyperadrenalism can occur via a number of conditions, more commonly as a result of pituitary tumor, and familial Cushing syndrome, leading to excess serum cortisol. In addition, the chronic use of systemic steroids may exogenously simulate this. The chronic elevated cortisol levels manifest with Cushingoid facial features resulting from fat redistribution, with the typical manifestation being a moon-shaped face and chubby cheeks. Intraorally, this condition may cause prominent bilateral indentation marks on the buccal mucosa and possible ulceration owing to trauma from the adjacent teeth.

Hypoadrenalism, also known as Addison's disease, results in decreased cortisol levels with reduction on the negative feedback on the pituitary gland, leading to increased secretion of pituitary adrenocorticotropic hormone cortisol. Owing to the molecular similarity between adrenocorticotropic hormone cortisol and melatonin-stimulating hormone, increased secretion of adrenocorticotropic hormone cortisol binds to the melanocortin receptors, and there is also an increase in release of other melanocyte-stimulating hormones. Oral mucosal hyperpigmentation can result, presenting as multiple, flat brownish plaques.

Thyroid Gland

Hypothyroidism in adults is reported to be associated with a burning sensation of the mouth, with the mechanism being unknown.[16] Congenital hypothyroidism, also known as congenital myxedema or cretinism, may result in macroglossia and delayed tooth eruption if not detected early and treated accordingly.

Growth Hormones

Growth hormone (GH)-releasing hormone from the hypothalamus promotes GH secretion from the pituitary, which in turn controls the growth of the entire body. Deficiency in GH results in dwarfism, whereas overproduction of GH during childhood results in gigantism, and overproduction in adults may result in acromegaly. Pituitary dwarfism may cause delayed growth of the skull and facial skeleton. In gigantism, growth disturbances usually present as a prognathic mandible, frontal bossing, dental malocclusion, and interdental spacing.[17] Radiologically, there may be hypercementosis of the roots, in which there is increased cementum, the outer layer of the roots and resultant change of morphology of the roots. Acromegaly in adults manifests as increased growth of the mandible, mandibular prognathism, spaced teeth, and macroglossia.[18] This condition may result in an Angle class III malocclusion (in which the mandible is in a protruded or in a prognathic relationship to the maxilla), and difficulty with biting or chewing. Other facial changes reported in the literature include thickened lips, protruded glabella, and increased anterior face height.

Diabetes

Periodontal disease is more common and severe in patients with uncontrolled diabetes (ie,: hemoglobin A1C of >7.0%). This has been extensively reported in type 2 diabetes and has less frequently been documented in type 1 diabetes. It has been reported that treatment for periodontitis has been noted to improve glycemic control and decrease hemoglobin A1c,[19] because it is postulated that the increased inflammation from each condition adversely affects the other.

Hyposalivation and sialodenosis (involving the minor salivary glands) may also present in diabetics. It has been suggested that neuropathy and microvascular abnormalities, with endothelial dysfunction and deterioration of microcirculation associated with diabetes, disrupts saliva flow and composition.[20]

Delayed wound healing is associated with poor glycemic control, and it is likely the result of microvasculature changes and compromised immune function. It may manifest as more severe oral ulcers and delayed postoperative wound healing.

Diabetic patients are more susceptible to oral candidiasis, most likely owing to the dry mouth, high levels of salivary glucose, salivary pH disorder, and impaired immune system.[21] Sensory disturbances in diabetes may include burning sensations, taste changes, and perioral neuropathies.

Parathyroid Gland

The parathyroid glands produce parathyroid hormone that, along with vitamin D, promote increased blood calcium levels. In hyperparathyroidism, there are mineral disturbances and generalized bone resorption, termed renal osteodystrophy. More recently, this syndrome was renamed chronic kidney disease–mineral and bone disorder.[22] This disease manifests in the jaw bones as loose trabeculation, blurring of the normal trabecular pattern, cortical thinning, and loss of the lamina dura, with tooth loosening

also having been reported.[13] A ground glass appearance is a radiologic change reflecting replacement of the normal jaw bone with poorly organized fibrotic tissue with irregular trabeculation, which in turn may result in jaw expansion.[23] Progression of bone resorption causes the formation of well-defined unilocular or multilocular radiolucencies, called brown tumors. Histologically, these lesions are similar to giant cell granulomas.[24] Dental pulp obliteration has been reported in individuals with secondary hyperparathyroidism.[24]

AUTOIMMUNE DISORDERS

Numerous autoimmune disorders have prominent oral manifestations, whether they are generalized systemic autoimmune disorders or those confined to the skin and mucosa. Some of these conditions, such as systemic lupus erythematosus, LP, pemphigus vulgaris, mucous membrane pemphigoid, and graft-versus-host disease are covered in elsewhere in this publication.

Sjögren's Syndrome

Sjögren's syndrome is an autoimmune rheumatic disease that primarily targets the salivary and lacrimal glands, but can also have a wide range of other organ specific and systemic manifestations. Worldwide, the overall prevalence of Sjögren's syndrome has been estimated to be 0.06%; however, owing to heterogeneity of studies and diagnostic criteria, it is in question with reports ranging from 0.01% to 3.00%.[24] The majority of orofacial manifestations (Sjögren's syndrome) are primarily a result of salivary gland hypofunction.

An increased risk of dental caries in patients has been associated with Sjögren's syndrome, with 1 study showing primary patients with Sjögren's syndrome having significantly higher measures of caries (decayed, missed, and filled surfaces), more missing teeth, and greater numbers of cariogenic and acidophilic microorganisms when compared with healthy controls.[25] Individuals with Sjögren's syndrome have a lower pH and buffer capacity when comparing findings with normal controls,[26] because phosphate, bicarbonate, and protein are responsible for the buffering capacity of saliva. Additionally, lessened stimulated salivary flow[27] has been associated with increased sugar clearance time, allowing cariogenic bacteria to more efficiently produce acid and thus increase levels of dental decay.[28] Conversely, there is no clear increase in the incidence or severity of periodontal disease in patients with Sjögren's syndrome.

Owing to hyposalivation, patients with Sjögren's syndrome may have dry and cracked lips with peeling, sores of the oral mucosa, and tongue depapillation, with a desiccated, deeply fissured, and sticky appearance (**Fig. 6**). Persons with Sjögren's syndrome have an increased occurrence of fungal infections (*Candida albicans*) than the general population,[29,30] because there is an inverse relationship between stimulated salivary flow rates and the level of *Candida* infection.[31]

Scleroderma

In scleroderma, or systemic sclerosis, abnormal amounts of dense collagen are deposited in most tissues of the body, with effects being most apparent in the skin. Microstomia, as characterized by a decreased mouth opening, is often seen as a result of collagen deposits in the perioral tissues (**Fig. 7**). Dysphagia occurs owing to the deposit of collagen in the lingual and esophageal submucosa, and a hypomobile tongue.

NUTRITIONAL DEFICIENCIES

Nutritional deficiencies can be due to impaired or decrease nutritional intake or due to impaired nutrient absorption. For example, individuals with autism may have food aversions and sensitivities, leading to decreased intake. Patients with alcohol dependence may have decreased intake, in addition to alcohol's direct effects on digestion, storage and metabolism of nutrients.

Vitamin A (Retinol) and Vitamin E Deficiency

Decreased intake and presumably deficiencies of vitamins A and E have been shown to be associated with increased severity of periodontal disease and deterioration of the dentition, as evidenced by the number of teeth, with the latter showing a temporal association of decline of the dentition with degree of nutrient intake.[32,33]

Vitamin B Deficiency

Among its many functions, vitamin B has a role in oral mucosal maintenance. The oral manifestations of iron, vitamin B_2 (riboflavin), B_3 (niacin), B_6 (pyridoxine), B_9 (folic acid; folate), and B_{12} (cobalamin) deficiencies are similar and include a smooth atrophic tongue (glossitis) with or without a burning sensation or pain (glossodynia), and cracking and fissuring of the lips (cheilitis), especially at the corners of the mouth (angular cheilitis). The smooth appearance of the tongue is caused by atrophy of the filiform papillae and, over time, the fungiform papillae may also degenerate. Vitamin B_6 (pyridoxine)

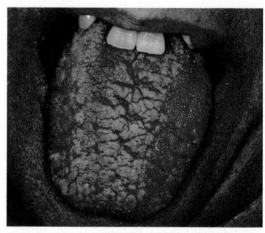

Fig. 6. Dry, fissured tongue in a patient with Sjögren's syndrome.

deficiency may present as seborrhea-like changes around the lips, nose and eyes. Vitamin B_7 (biotin) deficiency may cause periorofacial dermatitis with erythema and fine scaling around the mouth, eyes, nose, genitalia, and anus, but does not manifest in the oral mucosa. Insufficient intake of vitamin B_9 is significantly associated with increased severity of periodontal disease.[33] Vitamin B_9 and B_{12} deficiencies increase the tendency for recurrent aphthous ulcer with larger and clustered ulcers, in addition to altered taste and sensory changes in the oral tissues, typically a burning sensation in the tongue and the labial mucosa.[6]

Vitamin C (Ascorbic Acid) Deficiency

Vitamin C deficiency, also known as scurvy, may manifest as spontaneous gingival bleeding, and mucosal ulceration. Capillary fragility causes petechiae or more extensive ecchymosis. Additionally, a low intake of vitamin C increases the risk of

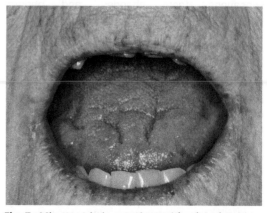

Fig. 7. Microstomia in a patient with scleroderma.

periodontal disease, with teeth mobility and loss reported.[15,34]

Vitamin K (Phylloquinone) Deficiency

Vitamin K is an essential cofactor in the coagulation cascade, and manifests clinically as mucosal or gingival bleeding. Vitamin K deficiency is often drug induced, but may occur in some pathologic conditions or due to drug interactions (see Bleeding Disorders, elsewhere in this article).

Iron Deficiency

The most common oral manifestation of iron deficiency is glossitis. As with vitamin B_{12} deficiency, it may be painful and present as loss of papillation, and may cause gustatory dysfunction.[35] Iron deficiency is a risk factor for candidal lesions, such as pseudomembranous oral candidiasis and angular cheilitis. In Plummer-Vinson syndrome (also known as Paterson-Kelly syndrome and sideropenic dysphagia and associated with iron deficiency), in addition to painful glossitis, there is dysphagia caused by esophageal webs. These patients are at risk of oral, hypopharyngeal, and esophageal squamous cell carcinoma.[36] Iron deficiency has also been significantly associated with increased severity of periodontal disease.

Zinc Deficiency

Zinc deficiency is associated with dysgeusia. Although previously being linked with oral aphthous ulcerations, 1 study indicated that decreased serum zinc levels had no impact on incidence and severity of oral aphthae.[37] In contrast, excessive application of topical zinc in denture adhesive has been reported to cause copper deficiency, which manifested itself as leukopenia, anemia, and neurologic changes to include perioral paresthesia and intraoral burning.[38]

INFECTIOUS DISEASES
Fungal Infections

The most common oral fungal infection is candidiasis owing to *C albicans* and, although it is considered a superficial oral infection, it can on rare occasions in immunosuppressed patients result in hematogenous spread if the mucosal barrier is compromised (eg, oral mucositis) or have respiratory spread if the patient is intubated. The 5 types of oral candidiasis are pseudomembranous, erythematous, rhomboid glossitis, candida leukoplakia (or hyperplastic), and angular cheilitis.

The most common presentation of oral candidiasis is the pseudomembranous type (**Fig. 8**), with multiple removable white plaques over an

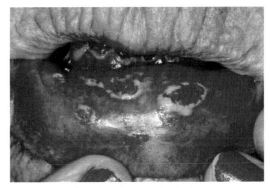

Fig. 8. Pseudomembranous candidiasis on the lower labial mucosa.

erythematous base, usually diagnosed clinically. Other presentations of oral candidiasis include erythematous patches on the palate (**Fig. 9**) or dorsum of the tongue, and erythema in the corners of the mouth (angular cheilitis) (**Fig. 10**). In long-standing oral candidiasis, white leukoplakia on the buccal mucosa or hypertrophic tissue on the midline dorsum or lateral borders of the tongue may be present (**Fig. 11**).

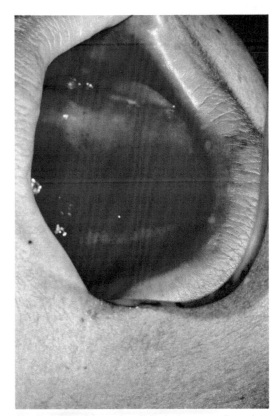

Fig. 9. Erythematous candidiasis seen on the palate and edentulous ridges of a patient who wears complete dentures, also known as denture stomatitis.

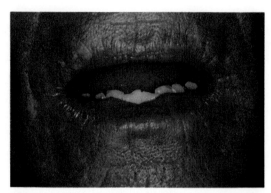

Fig. 10. Angular cheilitis as a result of fungal infection, presenting as erythema in the corners of the mouth.

Aspergillosis has been reported as the second most prevalent opportunistic fungal infection, although it is relatively rare in the oral cavity. Acquired by inhalation of spores, oral aspergillosis lesions are typically found in patients with cancer undergoing chemotherapy, found on the palate or posterior tongue, with lesions being yellow or black, with a necrotic ulcerated base. Mucormycosis is also an opportunistic infection that has rare occurrence in the orofacial region, with an association with diabetes mellitus, but also other immunosuppressive conditions such as solid organ (eg, renal) transplantation.[39] In both aspergillosis and mucormycosis, hematogenous spread may occur via after vessel penetration, thrombi formation (to include fatal cavernous sinus thrombosis), infarction, and tissue necrosis.[40]

Viral Infections

HSV is the most common oral viral infection, and oral presentations may be associated with a primary infection or systemic reactivation with break out in localized areas (eg, perioral or oral cavity), or more widespread involvement affecting multiple organs. Primary herpetic gingivostomatitis is an initial infection with HSV type I, and is characterized by erythematous, swollen, and painful gingiva. More common presentation of recurrent HSV infection is single or multiple pinhead-sized vesicles on the keratinized mucosa that quickly rupture into ulcers. However, in immunocompromised patients these lesions may be larger or coalesce and also involve the nonkeratinized mucosa (**Fig. 12**).

Varicella zoster virus, when it causes shingles (herpes zoster), presents similarly to HSV with vesicular eruptions, with the distinction that its distribution will is usually unilateral, correlating with a single trigeminal dermatome. The ophthalmic division (V1) of the trigeminal nerve is most affected,[41] but lesions can occur along the distribution of all 3 branches of the trigeminal nerve, both intraorally and extraorally. This finding is distinct from varicella (chicken pox), from initial acquisition of varicella zoster virus, which entails the onset of rashes and blisters throughout the body that does not follow a dermatome distribution. Oral lesions from varicella are typically raised papules that may form a shallow yellow or gray ulceration and are less painful than zoster lesions.

Cytomegalovirus is an opportunistic infection that may manifest as a nonspecific ulcer in immunocompromised patients such as those on immunosuppressants during cancer treatment or after transplantation, and in patients with AIDS. It is a relatively rare oral disease because all patients are screened for their serostatus and antiviral prophylaxis is standard practice in hematopoietic stem cell transplantation.

Coxsackie virus is responsible for hand, foot, and mouth disease, which typically occurs in children under 10 years of age and occasionally in

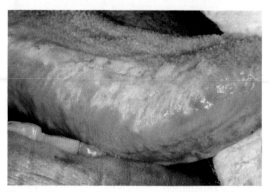

Fig. 11. Hyperplastic candidiasis on the lateral border of the tongue.

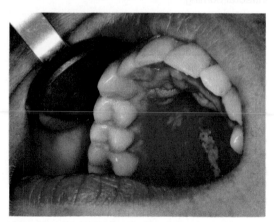

Fig. 12. Acute HSV infection involving the hard palate in an immunocompromised patient.

young adults. Blister-like rashes are seen on the hands, feet, and mouth, developing 1 to 2 days after initial symptoms of fever, poor appetite, sore throat, and runny nose. Herpangina, also caused by coxsackie virus, is characterized by small blisters primarily forming in the mouth and at the back of the throat, also affecting children.

Bacterial Infections

Bacterial infections of the oral mucosa are seen primarily in immunocompromised or immunosuppressed individuals. This pattern is different than common dental (odontogenic) infections, which commonly occur in immunocompetent individuals in addition to those with compromised or suppressed immune systems. They often present as a painful erosions or ulcerations, sometimes covered in a whitish fibrinous layer. The most common bacteria involved in infections in this patient population are enterococci. Gram-negative bacilli (*Pseudomonas aeruginosa*, *Klebsiella pneumoniae*) and gram-positive cocci (*Staphylococcus aureus*, *Staphylococcus epidermidis*, and *Streptococcus pyogenes*) are common micropathogens in immunosuppressed hematologic patients.[42]

Syphilis is a sexually transmitted disease caused by *Treponema pallidum*. It presents in 3 stages: primary, secondary, and tertiary syphilis. A primary lesion presents as a healing ulceration at the site of infection. Oral manifestations are less commonly the primary lesion, and more commonly at the secondary stage.[43] Various oral presentations include ulcerations, mucous patches, and maculopapular lesions (**Fig. 13**).

Tuberculosis has a rare occurrence in the oral cavity, with granulomatous lesions that have similar clinical appearance as syphilis, to include ulcerations, mucous patches, and even infrabony lesions seen as solitary radiolucencies. Oral lesions are usually secondarily inoculated owing to hematogenous spread or infected sputum.

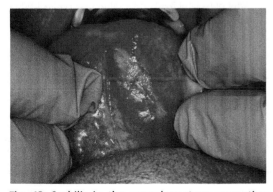

Fig. 13. Syphilis in the secondary stage presenting orally as a mucous patch on the ventral tongue.

NEUROLOGIC DISEASES

Orofacial manifestations of neurologic diseases include motor or sensory abnormalities that affect function or ability to perform routine oral hygiene measures.

Alzheimer Disease

The main orofacial complications in patients with Alzheimer's disease are due to the inability to self-care and carry out oral hygiene procedures, resulting in poor oral hygiene, an increased risk of dental caries, periodontal disease, and difficulty in wearing dentures.[44]

Stroke

Oral care in stroke can be challenging in patients that have loss and/or impairment of motor function. This difficulty is attributed to a lack of coordination, weakness, and cognitive problems. Therefore, their dentition and oral health condition is often compromised. In addition, stroke may result in sensory and motor deficits, weakness of facial muscles, and lack of tongue coordination, which may lead to food and debris accumulation going unnoticed by the patient. Conversely, a recent study found bacterial DNA from oral bacterial flora, namely *Streptococcus viridans*, in the thrombi of patients with acute ischemic stroke, raising a possible relationship between compromised oral flora in the progression of thrombotic cerebrovascular events.[45]

Parkinson's Disease

Orofacial manifestations in patients with Parkinson's disease include orofacial pain, oromandibular dystonias, increased caries and periodontal disease, sialorrhea, drooling, xerostomia, hyposalivation, bruxism (clenching and grinding), dysphagia, and dysgeusia.[46] Oral pain without any identifiable organic cause in these patients can be deemed neuropathic in origin, whereas dystonic type musculoskeletal pains can occur in the head and neck muscles.[47]

Multiple Sclerosis

As per the other conditions outlined in this article, motor function and ability to administer adequate self-care is a concern with individuals with multiple sclerosis (MS) owing to orofacial pain, spasticity, spasms, tremor, fatigue, depression, and disability. This finding can result in a compromised dental and oral health profile noted by increased burden of dental caries, gingivitis, and periodontitis.[48] Trigeminal neuralgia is reported in about 1.9% of cases of MS, but can be the first manifestation of MS in 0.3% of cases.[49] The tri-geminal neuralgia seen in MS patients can be bilateral, as opposed to conventional non–MS-associated cases in which it is unilateral. Sensory neuropathies secondary to MS can involve the mental nerve, causing numbness of the lower lip, and chin with or without pain. Facial paralysis can also occur in more advanced MS patients, occurring in up to 24.3% of cases.[50]

SUMMARY

Numerous systemic conditions can manifest in the oral and maxillofacial region and in the oral cavity, involving the dentition, soft tissues, bone, musculature and nerves. A coordinated approach between physicians and dentists in the diagnosis and management of these conditions is necessary to achieve optimal clinical outcomes.

DISCLOSURE

Dr M.T. Brennan is a consultant for Afyx. Dr S. Elad is a consultant for Falk Pharma.

REFERENCES

1. Di Fede O, Di Liberto C, Occhipinti G, et al. Oral manifestations in patients with gastro-oesophageal reflux disease: a single-center case-control study. J Oral Pathol Med 2008;37:336–40.
2. Mandel L, Vakkas J, Saqi A. Alcoholic (beer) sialosis. J Oral Maxillofac Surg 2005;63:402–5.
3. Guggenheimer J, Close JM, Eghtesad B. Sialadenosis in patients with advanced liver disease. Head Neck Pathol 2009;3(2):100–5.
4. Cassol-Spanemberg J, Rodríguez-de Rivera-Campillo ME, Otero-Rey EM, et al. Oral lichen planus and its relationship with systemic diseases. A review of evidence. J Clin Exp Dent 2018;10(9):e938–44.
5. Femiano F, Scully C. Functions of the cytokines in relation oral lichen planus-hepatitis C. Med Oral Patol Oral Cir Bucal 2005;10:e40–4.
6. Sun A, Chen HM, Cheng SJ, et al. Significant association of deficiencies of hemoglobin, iron, vitamin B12, and folic acid and high homocysteine level with recurrent aphthous stomatitis. J Oral Pathol Med 2015;44(4):300–5.
7. Samaranayake LP. Superficial oral fungal infections. Curr Opin Dent 1991;1(4):415–22.
8. Hazza'a AM, Al-Jamal G. Radiographic features of the jaws and teeth in thalassaemia major. Dentomaxillofac Radiol 2006;35(4):283–8.
9. Helmi N, Bashir M, Shireen A, et al. Thalassemia review: features, dental considerations and management. Electron Physician 2017;9(3):4003–8.
10. Guimarães T, Ferreira-Cabrini M, Quaglio C, et al. Temporomandibular disorder: prevalence among hemophiliac patients. International Journal of Odontostomatology 2015;9:295–300.
11. Scully C, et al. Oral lesions indicative of plasminogen deficiency (hypoplasminogenemia). Oral Surg Oral Med Oral Pathol Oral Radiol Endod 2001;91(3):334–7.
12. Chi AC, et al. Pseudomembranous disease (ligneous inflammation) of the female genital tract, peritoneum, gingiva, and paranasal sinuses associated with plasminogen deficiency. Ann Diagn Pathol 2009;13(2):132–9.
13. Silva TD, Ferreira CB, Leite GB, et al. Oral manifestations of lymphoma: a systematic review. Ecancermedicalscience 2016;10:665.
14. Balasubramaniam R, Goradia A, Turner LN, et al. Burkitt lymphoma of the oral cavity: an atypical presentation. Oral Surg Oral Med Oral Pathol Oral Radiol Endod 2009;107(2):240–5.
15. Hicks J, Flaitz CM. Langerhans cell histiocytosis: current insights in a molecular age with emphasis on clinical oral and maxillofacial pathology practice. Oral Surg Oral Med Oral Pathol Oral Radiol Endod 2005;100(2 Suppl):S42–66.
16. Femiano F, Lanza A, Buonaiuto C, et al. Burning mouth syndrome and burning mouth in hypothyroidism: proposal for a diagnostic and therapeutic protocol. Oral Surg Oral Med Oral Pathol Oral Radiol Endod 2008;105(1):e22–7.
17. Shafer GW, Hine MK, Levy BM, editors. A textbook of oral pathology. 4th edition. Hong Kong: Harcourt Brace Asia Inc; 1994. p. 654–7. Oral aspects of metabolic disease.
18. Kreitschmann-Andermahr I, et al. Oro-dental pathologies in acromegaly. Endocrine 2018;60(2):323–8.
19. Preshaw PM, Bissett SM. Periodontitis and diabetes. Br Dent J 2019;227(7):577–84.
20. von Bultzingslowen I, et al. Salivary dysfunction associated with systemic diseases: systematic review and clinical management recommendations. Oral Surg Oral Med Oral Pathol Oral Radiol Endod 2007;103(Suppl):S57.e1-15.
21. Kadir T, Pisiriciler R, Akyüz S, et al. Mycological and cytological examination of oral candidal carriage in diabetic patients and non-diabetic control subjects: thorough analysis of local aetiologic and systemic factors. J Oral Rehabil 2002;29(5):452–7.
22. Chapter 1: introduction and definition of CKD-MBD and the development of the guideline statements. Kidney Int 2009;76113:S3.
23. Pontes FSC, et al. Oral and maxillofacial manifestations of chronic kidney disease-mineral and bone disorder: a multicenter retrospective study. Oral Surg Oral Med Oral Pathol Oral Radiol 2018;125(1):31–43.

24. Maciel G, Crowson CS, Matteson EL, et al. Prevalence of primary Sjögren's syndrome in a US population-based cohort. Arthritis Care Res (Hoboken) 2017;69(10):1612–6.

25. Pedersen AM, Bardow A, Nauntofte B. Salivary changes and dental caries as potential oral markers of autoimmune salivary gland dysfunction in primary Sjogren's syndrome. BMC Clin Pathol 2005;5(1):4.

26. Soto-Rojas AE, Kraus A. The oral side of Sjögren syndrome. Diagnosis and treatment. A review. Arch Med Res 2002;33:95–106.

27. Bardow A, ten Cate JM, Nauntofte B, et al. Effect of unstimulated saliva flow rate on experimental root caries. Caries Res 2003;37:232–6.

28. Leone CW, Oppenheim FG. Physical and chemical aspects of saliva as indicators of risk for dental caries in humans. J Dent Educ 2001;65:1054–62.

29. MacFarlane TW, Mason DK. Changes in the oral flora in Sjögren's syndrome. J Clin Pathol 1974;27:416–9.

30. Radfar L, Shea Y, Fischer SH, et al. Fungal load and candidiasis in Sjögren's syndrome. Oral Surg Oral Med Oral Pathol Oral Radiol Endod 2003;96:283–7.

31. Tapper-Jones L, Aldred M, Walker DM. Prevalence and intraoral distribution of Candida albicans in Sjögren's syndrome. J Clin Pathol 1980;33:282–7.

32. Luo PP, Xu HS, Chen YW, et al. Periodontal disease severity is associated with micronutrient intake. Aust Dent J 2018;63(2):193–201.

33. Iwasaki M, et al. Longitudinal association of dentition status with dietary intake in Japanese adults aged 75 to 80 years. J Oral Rehabil 2016;43(10):737–44.

34. Nishida M, et al. Dietary vitamin C and the risk for periodontal disease. J Periodontol 2000;71(8):1215–23.

35. Wu YC, Wang YP, Chang JY, et al. Oral manifestations and blood profile in patients with iron deficiency anemia. J Formos Med Assoc 2014;113(2):83–7.

36. Samad A, Mohan N, Balaji RV, et al. Oral manifestations of Plummer-Vinson syndrome: a classic report with literature review. J Int Oral Health 2015;7(3):68–71.

37. Ślebioda Z, Krawiecka E, Szponar E, et al. Evaluation of serum zinc levels in patients with recurrent aphthous stomatitis (RAS). BMC Oral Health 2017;17(1):158.

38. Prasad R, Hawthorne B, Durai D, et al. Zinc in denture adhesive: a rare cause of copper deficiency in a patient on home parenteral nutrition. BMJ Case Rep 2015;2015. bcr2015211390.

39. Deepa A, Nair BJ, Sivakumar T, et al. Uncommon opportunistic fungal infections of oral cavity: a review. J Oral Maxillofac Pathol 2014;18(2):235–43.

40. Dreizen S. Oral complications of cancer therapies: description and incidence of oral complications. NCI Monogr 1990;9:11–5.

41. Klasser GD, Ahmed AS. How to manage acute herpes zoster affecting trigeminal nerves. J Can Dent Assoc 2014;80:e42.

42. Khan SA, Wingard JR. Infection and mucosal injury in cancer treatment. J Natl Cancer Inst Monogr 2001;(29):31–6.

43. Little JW. Syphilis: an update. Oral Surg Oral Med Oral Pathol Oral Radiol Endod 2005;100(1):3–9.

44. Mancini M, Grappasonni I, Scuri S, et al. Oral health in Alzheimer's disease: a review. Curr Alzheimer Res 2010;7(4):368–73.

45. Patrakka O, Pienimäki JP, Tuomisto S, et al. Oral bacterial signatures in cerebral thrombi of patients with acute ischemic stroke treated with thrombectomy. J Am Heart Assoc 2019;8(11):e012330.

46. Nakayama Y, Washio M, Mori M. Oral health conditions in patients with Parkinson's disease. J Epidemiol 2004;14(5):143–50.

47. Ford B, Louis ED, Greene P, et al. Oral and genital pain syndromes in Parkinson's disease. Mov Disord 1996;11(4):421–6.

48. Fiske J, Griffiths J, Thompson S. Multiple sclerosis and oral care. Dent Update 2002;29(6):273–83.

49. Isselbacher KJ, Wilson JD, Braunwald E, et al. 13th edition. Harrison's principles of internal medicine, vol. 2. New York: McGraw-Hill; 1994. p. 2287–94.

50. Fukazawa T, Moriwaka F, Hamada K, et al. Facial palsy in multiple sclerosis. J Neurol 1997;244:631–3.

Oral Potentially Malignant Disorders and Oral Cavity Cancer

David Ojeda, DDS[a], Michaell A. Huber, DDS[b], Alexander R. Kerr, DDS, MSD[c],*

KEYWORDS

• Oral cavity • Cancer • Potentially malignant disorders • Leukoplakia • Erythroplakia

KEY POINTS

• The Surveillance, Epidemiology, and End Results program from the National Cancer Institute reports that oral and pharyngeal cancer cases have been increasing over the past decade, and this is largely related to an increase in cancers involving oropharyngeal subsites.
• Early detection of oral cavity cancers is commensurate with improved survival, and opportunistic screening by trained clinicians to detect oral cavity cancer and oral potentially malignant disorders is recommended by the American Dental Association and the American Academy of Oral Medicine.
• A visual and tactile oral examination followed by biopsy with histologic evaluation of lesions detected that meet the clinical criteria for oral potentially malignant disorders remains the gold standard to establish a definitive diagnosis.
• The evidence-based management of patients with oral cavity cancer requires a multidisciplinary team and treatment modalities, including surgery, radiation, chemotherapy, and immunotherapy, as dictated by staging. The management of patients with oral epithelial dysplasia is not well defined.

INTRODUCTION

Cancer is the second leading cause of death in the United States, and oral and pharyngeal cancers represent 3% of all cancers diagnosed annually in the United States.[1] Traditionally, oral cavity and pharyngeal cancers have been grouped together because of their anatomic location; however, research spanning the last 2 decades has shown significant differences in the etiopathogenesis of cancers affecting these subsites. In particular, the identification of oncogenic human papillomavirus infection as a major risk factor for oropharyngeal cancer makes it distinct from oral cavity cancers (OCC), which are largely related to lifestyle factors, such as tobacco and/or heavy alcohol use.[2] However, there remains some confusion about these distinctions, and the term "oral cancer" is often used erroneously to collectively represent these 2 subsites. This review focuses on OCC and oral potentially malignant disorders (OPMD). Readers interested in learning more about oropharyngeal cancer are recommended to read excellent reviews on this topic.[3,4]

The most common type of cancer affecting the oral cavity is squamous cell carcinoma (herein abbreviated with the acronym OSCC), and most OSCCs are preceded by OPMDs, a group of oral mucosal lesions and conditions that confer an increased risk for malignant transformation.[5] The authors describe several OPMDs, including leukoplakia, erythroplakia, oral lichen planus (OLP), oral submucous fibrosis (OSF), actinic cheilitis, and

[a] Department of Comprehensive Dentistry, University of Texas Health Science Center San Antonio, School of Dentistry, 7703 Floyd Curl Drive, office 2.565U, San Antonio, TX 78229-3900, USA; [b] Department of Comprehensive Dentistry, University of Texas Health Science Center San Antonio, School of Dentistry, 7703 Floyd Curl Drive, San Antonio, TX 78229-3900, USA; [c] Department of Oral & Maxillofacial Pathology, Radiology and Medicine, New York University College of Dentistry, 345 East 24th Street, Room 813C, New York, NY 10010, USA
* Corresponding author.
E-mail address: ark3@nyu.edu

Dermatol Clin 38 (2020) 507–521
https://doi.org/10.1016/j.det.2020.05.011
0733-8635/20/© 2020 Elsevier Inc. All rights reserved.

proliferative verrucous leukoplakia (PVL). The early detection of OSCCs and OPMDs is critical to improving patient outcomes. OSCCs and OPMDs may be discovered during routine oral examinations in primary or secondary care settings. Dermatologists are experts in the diagnosis of cutaneous malignancies and dermatologic disorders overlapping with oral mucosal diseases; therefore, by performing opportunistic oral examinations, they have the potential to increase the number of patients who otherwise do not receive an adequate examination. This review serves as an overview of the current diagnosis and management of OSCCs and OPMDs.

EPIDEMIOLOGY IN NORTH AMERICA
Oral Cavity Cancer

The Surveillance, Epidemiology, and End Results (SEER) program in the United States reports epidemiologic data for oral cavity, lip, and pharyngeal subsites (oropharynx, nasopharynx, and hypopharynx) in aggregate. The age-adjusted incidence for the aggregate of oral cavity and pharyngeal cancers (2012–2016) is approximately 11.3/100,000 and has been increasing by an average of 0.8% over the last decade.[6] Incidence of oral cavity and oropharyngeal subsites comprises 6.1 and 2.4 per 100,000, respectively, collectively translating to approximately 75% of all oral cavity and pharyngeal cancers (54% and 21%, respectively).[6] Mortality has remained stable at approximately 2.5/100,000, and the age-adjusted 5-year survival rate is 65.3%. In 2019, this translated to an estimated 53,000 cases, and 10,800 deaths.[6] Greater than 90% of these cancers are squamous cell carcinomas (SCC), and the remaining 10% comprise salivary gland malignancies, sarcomas, myeloproliferative cancers, and mucosal melanomas; these will not be covered in this review.

Oropharynx Cancer

Recent data show that more than 18,000 oropharynx cancers are diagnosed annually in the United States (of which approximately 70% are attributed to human papillomavirus infection) with an average annual increase of 2.7% since 1999.[7]

Oral Potentially Malignant Disorders

OPMDs are defined as oral mucosal lesions and conditions with unclear cause that have malignant potential. Examples include leukoplakia, erythroplakia,[5] OLP, OSF, PVL, and actinic cheilitis.[8] Other disorders with increased malignant potential include oral graft-versus-host disease,[9] Li-Fraumeni syndrome,[10] dyskeratosis congenita,[11] and Fanconi anemia.[12] The reported overall prevalence of OPMDs is 4.4%.[13] Leukoplakia is the most commonly observed OPMD, with prevalence estimates of 1.7% to 2.7%,[14] and an annual risk for malignant transformation of 2% to 3%.[15] Erythroplakia is comparatively rare with prevalence estimates of 0.02% to 0.83% and usually represents high-grade dysplasia or SCC at discovery.[16] If not malignant at baseline, erythroplakia has a malignant transformation rate of 14% to 50%.[17] OPMDs that undergo biopsy may demonstrate histologic evidence of oral epithelial dysplasia (OED). For either leukoplakia or erythroplakia, the higher the grade of OED, the greater the risk for malignant transformation.[18] OPMDs with moderate/severe dysplasia confer more than twice the risk for malignant transformation than those that exhibit mild dysplasia.[19] It is important to note that a small fraction of OPMDs without dysplasia can harbor molecular alterations[20] and progress to cancer.[21]

The malignant potential of OLP and other lichenoid conditions remains a topic of debate. For OLP, a large metaanalysis determined a pooled risk for malignant transformation of 1.14% (95% confidence interval: 0.84–1.49). The risk was highest for the erosive lichen planus subtype involving the tongue followed by the buccal mucosa.[22] OSF, an inflammatory disease characterized by progressive stiffening of the oral mucosa, is commonly observed in South East Asia in patients who use areca nut products.[23] The presence of OED at discovery is approximately 25%, and the malignant transformation rate varies from 3% to 19%.[23,24]

PVL is characterized by multifocal leukoplakia occurring predominantly in older women, irrespective of conventional risk factors.[25] Patients with PVL have a high risk for malignant transformation (60% to 100%), frequent recurrences after total excision (87% to 100%), and high mortalities (30% to 50%).[26]

Actinic cheilitis results from UV radiation to the lips and is most commonly observed in men older than 50 years of age. The estimated malignant transformation ranges from 10% to 30%,[27] and most SCCs of the lip are preceded by actinic cheilitis.[28,29]

The International Agency for Research on Cancer has identified tobacco (in all forms),[30,31] alcohol use,[32] areca nut use,[33] low socioeconomic status,[34] and poor diet[35] as independent risk factors for OSCC. There is also limited evidence identifying poor oral hygiene,[36] and periodontitis[37] as possible risk factors. The risk factors for OPMDs and OSCCs are essentially the same.[38,39]

PATHOGENESIS AND NATURAL HISTORY

Most OSCCs develop following a stepwise accumulation of genetic and epigenetic alterations. These alterations are typically the result of long-term exposure to the aforementioned carcinogenic risk factors. However, OSCCs arise from a heterogeneous genetic and epigenetic landscape, and as such, the natural history of their development and evolution (ie, metastasis) is variable. A small fraction of OSCCs develop de novo, but most are preceded by OPMDs, and the propensity for malignant progression of these OPMDs is difficult to predict. At the molecular level, clones of epithelial cells are subjected to continued genetic and epigenetic alterations (eg, mutations in important oncogenes and tumor suppressor genes, such as *p53*).[40] The cumulative effect of these disruptions over time eventually becomes irreversible, resulting in malignancy. The concept of "field cancerization" infers tissues at risk contain numerous altered clones of epithelial cells in different phases of malignant progression.[41] Ongoing research into the molecular pathogenesis of OSCCs has identified numerous biomarkers associated with tumor initiation and progression, offering the hope of developing a personalized approach to OSCC management.[40] Mehanna and colleagues[42] reported that OPMDs with high grades of dysplasia are more than twice as likely to undergo malignant transformation (mild/moderate 10.3% vs severe 24.1%). In the molecular arena, the loss of heterozygosity at key chromosomal loci (eg, 3p14, 9p21) and DNA ploidy are 2 examples of OPMDs malignant transformation predictive biomarkers that have been validated in longitudinal studies,[42,43] although there are no commercial tests available yet. Unfortunately, the application of precision medicine has thus far not benefited patients with OSCCs and OPMDs.

For patients with OPMDs, there are valuable clinical and histopathologic predictive factors for clinicians to consider. Lesions diagnosed with high-grade dysplasia are at greater risk for malignant transformation. The risk of malignant transformation is greater if the patient is over the age of 45 years, a woman, and a non-smoker. Lesions occurring on floor of the mouth, ventrolateral tongue, retromolar area, and soft palate are at higher risk of malignant transformation. Lesions that are greater than 200 mm^2 and/or nonhomogeneous are at greater risk for malignant transformation.[44]

SCREENING
Types of Screening

Screening for OCC or OPMDs is strictly defined as the organized application of a screening test to a large population that is asymptomatic and apparently free of disease in order to identify those who may have OCC or OPMDs.[45] Such "organized" screening is distinct from the typical "opportunistic" screening or "case finding" that a patient might undergo during a routine visit to a dental or medical practice.

Screening Guidelines in the United States

Screening for the early detection of both OCC and OPMDs can reduce the cancer-specific morbidity and mortality.[46] Nevertheless, very few countries have adopted national oral cancer screening programs because of the relative rarity of the disease, the lack of knowledge of the natural history of the disease, and the lack of evidence on the efficacy and cost-effectiveness of different screening methods.[47] Lack of evidence regarding the benefits and harms of screening for OCC in asymptomatic adults in primary care settings was also reported by the US Preventive Service Task Force.[48] However, opportunistic screening for OCC and OPMDs during visits to the dentist (or expert medical professionals) is recommended by the American Dental Association and the American Academy of Oral Medicine.[49] OCC opportunistic screening is not an isolated event but rather 1 component of the comprehensive head and neck examination and represents an opportunity to assess any oral abnormalities, whether neoplastic, infectious, reactive/inflammatory, or developmental.[50] In a primary care dental setting, such opportunistic screenings should be performed not only during the new patient examination but also at recalls, and emergency or problem-focused visits for all patients, but particularly in those who use tobacco or who consume alcohol heavily. Dermatologists with experience in the examination of the oral cavity are encouraged to perform opportunistic oral examinations, or otherwise recommend patients seek such an examination at a dental office.

CLINICAL ASSESSMENT AND DIAGNOSIS ORAL CAVITY CANCER AND ORAL POTENTIALLY MALIGNANT DISORDERS
Clinical Assessment

A variety of conditions affecting the oral cavity can present with overlapping signs and symptoms; therefore, a thorough history and comprehensive visual and tactile oral cavity examination should be performed.[51] While eliciting the history, clinicians must pay special attention to presenting symptoms, and the presence of established risk factors for OCC and OPMDs, such as history of habits (especially the use of alcohol and tobacco), underlying medical conditions or medications leading to immunosuppression, a past history of cancer, and other environmental exposures.[52] Relative to symptoms, a patient's initial complaint may be variable and may include one or more of the following: a sensation of an altered mucosa, a lesion or sore that has not healed, abnormal oral bleeding, a lump in the neck, and changes in swallowing or oral function, or pain. Pain may be experienced particularly during oral function (known as mechanical allodynia) and may indicate OCC irrespective of the clinical staging.[53] Leukoplakia and erythroplakia are typically not painful. Depending on the severity of the disease, patients with OSF and OLP may complain of oral burning and sensitivity to acidic and spicy foods, beverages, or oral hygiene products.

The physical examination includes a visual and tactile assessment of extraoral and intraoral structures within the head and neck area. The extraoral examination begins with a visual inspection of the head and neck to detect swellings, asymmetries, discolorations, and abnormal skin changes or lesions. OCC typically metastasizes via the regional lymphatic system and can manifest as cervical lymphadenopathy as palpably firm, nontender, and in some cases, nonmoveable or fixed lymph nodes. Salivary gland and thyroid malignancies may also be detected, and palpation of these structures is also necessary. Clinicians may also perform a cranial nerve examination to evaluate patients for neurologic changes that may be associated with OCC, particularly those in advanced stages. Dysesthesia, paresthesia, or loss of motor function may be symptoms indicating tumor growth owing to nerve compression or invasion.

The intraoral examination is intended to differentiate normal from abnormal mucosa and requires a systematic approach. To properly perform an intraoral examination, a bright light source and a tongue depressor and a piece of gauze are recommended. The intraoral examination involves the inspection of all visible intraoral surfaces, including the oropharynx (**Fig. 1**). All intraoral structures should be closely examined in a consistent systematic fashion looking for abnormal changes in color or texture that might suggest pathologic condition. In addition, palpation of the lips, vestibules, hard palate, tongue, and floor of the mouth will help detect submucosal nodules or masses that may not be visible on the surface. Palpation provides valuable clinical information regarding the consistency and size of the lesion found. Induration, the term used to describe the palpable firmness associated with lesions that have invaded deeper structures, is an ominous feature that may be suggestive of OCC. Similarly, in patients with symptoms of pain, palpation may facilitate the identification of the site of pain. **Table 1** is a

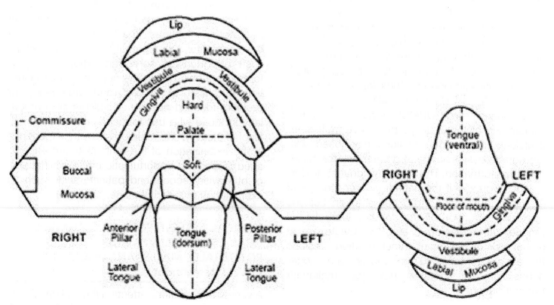

Fig. 1. Oral cavity map. (*From* Laronde, D. M., Williams, P. M., Hislop, T. G., et al (2014). Influence of fluorescence on screening decisions for oral mucosal lesions in community dental practices. Journal of oral pathology & medicine, 43(1), 7-13 with permission.)

Table 1
Extraoral and intraoral examination checklist

Extraoral	Intraoral

Visual inspection:
  Facial skin (discoloration, changes in
    surface, scar tissue)
  Lesions
  Facial asymmetry (swelling, masses)
  Salivary gland enlargement (parotid)
  Neurologic deficiencies (ptosis, facial palsy)
	Visual inspection:
	  Lips (labial mucosa, commissures)
	  Buccal mucosa
	  Vestibule (maxillary and mandibular)
	  Gingiva (facial, buccal, palatine, lingual,
	    attached, marginal)
	  Hard and soft palate
	Oropharynx:
	• Uvula
	• Anterior and posterior tonsillar pillars
	• Palatine tonsils

Palpate:
Lymph nodes
• Preauricular and postauricular, occipital,
  mastoid, submandibular, submental, and
  the anterior and posterior superficial cervi-
  cal lymph nodes
Glands
• Major salivary glands (parotid, submandib-
  ular, and sublingual)
• Thyroid gland
Temporomandibular joint (TMJ)/masticatory
  muscles (temporalis, masseter)
	Palpate:
	  Lips
	  Vestibules (maxillary and mandibular)
	  Hard palate
	  Tongue (ventral, dorsal, and lateral borders)
	  Floor of the mouth

checklist that summarizes the intraoral and extraoral structures that should be evaluated. A synthesis of history and examination findings leads a clinician toward a diagnosis. When a single clinical diagnosis cannot be made, the clinician should develop a differential diagnosis containing a list of 2 or more potential diagnoses ordered with the most likely diagnosis on the top. To establish a definitive diagnosis, further testing, such as tissue biopsy, imaging, or laboratory tests, may be indicated.

Clinical Features: Oral Cavity Cancer

OSCCs are epithelial-derived cancers and comprise more than 90% of all OCC. They can arise from any mucosal surface of the mouth, affecting most commonly the anterior two-thirds of the tongue, followed by the floor of the mouth, lips, buccal mucosa, gingiva, and palate.[54] OSCCs can present with variable clinical features. These features may include cancers that are exophytic (ie, growing off of the surface) (**Fig. 2**) versus ulcerative (ie, invading below the surface) (**Fig. 3**). OSCCs may appear red, white, mixed red and white, and/or as ulcerated lesions (some cancers can also present as a solitary ulcer without red and white changes), and the surface can appear granular, nodular, or verrucous (**Fig. 4**). Some

cancerous lesions may be friable (ie, bleed easily upon slight provocation). Other less common OCC, such as salivary gland malignancies, may present as submucosal nodules or masses with or without surface ulceration. The clinical presentation and the associated symptoms will depend on the stage OF disease, the location of the lesion, and the underlying genetic/epigenetic alterations driving carcinogenesis.

Early cancers tend to have more subtle signs compared with more advanced disease, which may be deeply ulcerated, grossly exophytic, and associated with regional lymphadenopathy and alteration of oral function (ie, dysphagia, odynophagia, trismus, difficulty chewing, or dysphonia).[55] Of interest, the presence of pain is variable at the time of presentation and does not necessarily correlate with stage of disease (eg, early-stage OCC can demonstrate pain, particularly mechanical allodynia).[53]

Clinical Features: Oral Potentially Malignant Disorders

Leukoplakia and erythroplakia are clinical diagnoses. Leukoplakia is defined as a white mucosal patch that cannot be defined as any other disorder and carries an increased risk of malignant transformation.[5] Two clinical subtypes of leukoplakia have

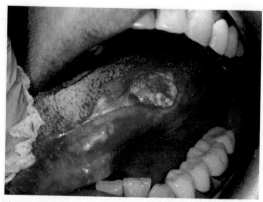

Fig. 2. Exophytic lesion on left lateral border of the tongue consistent with OSCC.

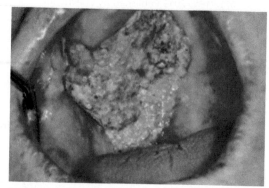

Fig. 4. Granular, nodular/verrucous lesion consistent with OSCC.

been described. Homogenous leukoplakia presents as a uniformly white patch that may express cracks and fissures on the surface (**Fig. 5**), whereas nonhomogenous leukoplakia presents with mixed colors (white and red) and different patterns on the surface topography (papillary, nodular, or verrucous) (**Fig. 6**).[18] Experts agree that nonhomogenous leukoplakia carries a higher risk of being malignant at baseline or of undergoing malignant transformation.[18] The most commonly affected sites for leukoplakia are the buccal mucosa (25%), followed by the gingiva (20%), and ventral tongue and floor of the mouth (10%).[56] Leukoplakia is considered a dynamic lesion in that it can progress, or in some cases regress, and therefore, the clinical presentation can vary in size, color, and surface topography over time.[18]

PVL predominantly occur in women and are associated with a high risk for progression and malignant transformation (>70%).[26] Clinically, patients demonstrate a slow evolution from unifocal to multifocal leukoplakias, most frequently involving the gingiva and buccal mucosa. Often the lesions present with a verrucous surface, although some patients exhibit no verrucous features, and new diagnostic criteria have been proposed[57] (**Fig. 7**).

Erythroplakia is described as a bright red plaque with a velvety surface. Erythroplakia usually presents as an asymptomatic lesion affecting most commonly the soft palate, floor of the mouth, and buccal mucosa (**Fig. 8**). OLP can present with a variety of clinical presentations. Reticular lichen planus presents as white, small papules with a lacy pattern known as Wickham striae and tends to be asymptomatic. Atrophic and erosive lichen planus presents with various degrees of inflammation causing thinning of the epithelium, which clinically presents as areas of mucosal erosions and ulcerations that frequently are surrounded by striae and produce erythema, pain, soreness, and bleeding upon manipulation. Lichen

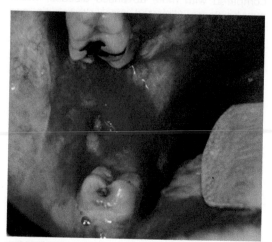

Fig. 3. Solitary ulcer on right retromolar area consistent with OSCC.

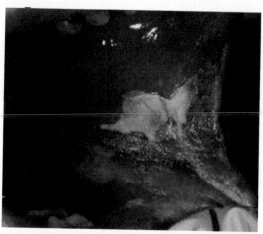

Fig. 5. Homogeneous leukoplakia on left anterior buccal mucosa.

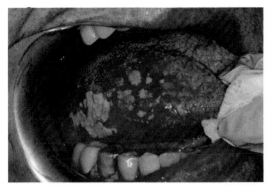

Fig. 6. Nonhomogeneous leukoplakia (erythroleukoplakia) on right lateral and dorsal tongue. Note the combination of colors throughout the lesion (whitered) and the different patterns of surface topography.

planus typically presents as symmetric, bilateral lesions affecting the buccal mucosa, tongue, and gingiva (**Fig. 9**).

OSF occurs in patients with a history of chewing betel quid and related areca nut products (largely in patients from South Asia). Patients initially experience a burning sensation and intolerance for spicy foods. Over time, they develop a progressive fibrosis involving the buccal mucosa, retromolar area, and soft palate, and this can result in severe limitation in mouth opening and may affect speech.[58]

Actinic cheilitis more frequently affects the lower lip and is typically asymptomatic. Initially, it may present as dry and scaly lips. More advanced stages may exhibit areas of erosions, and loss of the vermillion border definition with an opalescent appearance and the presence of white or gray plaques[59] (**Fig. 10**).

Adjunctive Techniques

The presence of small, subtle, or early-stage lesions, in conjunction with the broad spectrum of clinical presentations of OCC and OPMDs, represents a diagnostic challenge. The conventional visual and tactile oral examination is limited in its inability to discriminate benign lesions from premalignant or malignant lesions.[60] Several adjunctive techniques have been developed in an effort to aid the clinician to detect lesions during an opportunistic screening examination (screening adjunct), to facilitate the risk stratification of lesions detected during examination (diagnostic adjunct), or to determine the malignant potential of a lesion (predictive adjunct).[61] Products currently available to clinicians in the US marketplace include optical aids, such as those based on differences in tissue autofluorescence or tissue reflectance in OSCCs and OPMDs

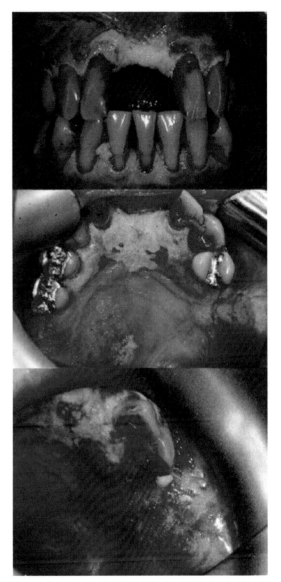

Fig. 7. PVL. Note multifocal leukoplakia in the 2 top images. Over time, progression of disease ultimately led to malignant transformation of the upper left maxillary alveolus.

(analogous to the Wood's lamp used in dermatology), vital staining with toluidine blue, cytopathologic platforms, and most recently, salivary diagnostics. Although most of these techniques have shown proof of concept, the evidence to support their use is still low.[50] These techniques should not be considered a substitute for the conventional diagnostic pathway (ie, biopsy with histopathologic analysis) to establish a definitive diagnosis. Clinicians who perform these techniques should undergo training and carefully interpret the results in the context of the patient's medical history and other clinical findings.

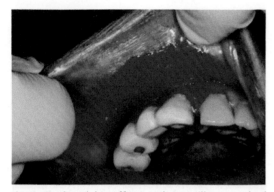

Fig. 8. Erythroplakia affecting the maxillary attached gingiva, maxillary vestibule, and upper labial mucosa.

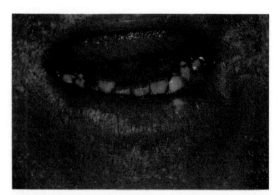

Fig. 10. Lower lip with signs of actinic cheilitis. Note loss of definition of the vermillion border, and white patch on lower left vermillion.

Biopsy Site Selection

Biopsy with histopathologic analysis remains the "gold standard" for the diagnosis of OSCCs and OPMDs. Because of the variety of clinical presentations of OCC and OPMDs, along with the potential for variable histopathology within the field of a single lesion, the selection of a representative area of the lesion can be challenging, even for the expert clinician. Before biopsy, consider the size, anatomic location, and clinical appearance of the lesion. From a baseline diagnostic perspective, excisional biopsies are indicated for small, well-demarcated lesions that have a low index of suspicion for malignancy. Otherwise, single or multiple incisional biopsies may be procured. If present, areas of induration are highly suspicious for a malignancy, and these areas should be biopsied first. Because depth of invasion (DOI) is a prognostic factor for OSCC, it is important to provide deeper biopsy specimens that allow this determination.[62] Erythema and ulceration are signs that suggest higher-grade histopathology compared with white areas. Large and nonhomogenous lesions may exhibit different histologic features in different areas; therefore, multiple specimens may be required.

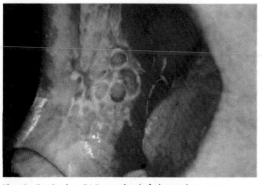

Fig. 9. Reticular OLP on the left buccal mucosa.

Histology

OSCCs typically, but not exclusively, originate from dysplastic epithelium. Atypical epithelial cells may exhibit enlarged and hyperchromatic nuclei, increased nuclear-to-cytoplasmic ratio, pleomorphic cells, dyskeratosis, and increased and abnormal mitosis.[63] The number and distribution of atypical epithelial cells within the epithelium determine the degree of dysplasia (mild, moderate, or severe). The aggregation of epithelial atypical cells can result in architectural changes in the tissue, and such changes include bulbous rete ridges, loss of polarity, keratin pearls, and loss of typical cell cohesion.[63] All these histologic findings reflect the biological alterations in the cells that affect their maturation pattern in the epithelium. Atypical epithelial cells penetrating into the underlying connective tissue is called invasion, and this feature distinguishes carcinoma in situ from invasive carcinomas. As infiltration of the cancer proceeds, there is an increased risk for invasion of lymphatics, blood vessels, nerve, and other surrounding tissue. Tumor invasion plays a significant role in disease prognosis.[62] Mandibular bone invasion is associated with aggressive tumor behavior and increased risk of death, whereas lymphatic and nerve invasion increases the risk of metastasis and recurrence.[64,65]

IMAGING FOR ORAL CAVITY CANCER

Imaging is used to determine the extension of the primary tumor, to assess regional lymph nodes, and to evaluate distant metastasis. Cross-sectional imaging, such as computed tomography (CT) with intravenous (IV) contrast and MRI with IV contrast, will provide information regarding the size and the relationship of the tumor to other anatomic structures. CT scans can precisely detect cortical erosions, whereas MRI is more sensitive for bone marrow involvement.[66] Distant metastases are usually assessed with a PET scan because of its sensitivity in detecting metabolic activity. Often, a panoramic radiograph is obtained to evaluate the overall dental health of the patient before cancer treatment (**Fig. 11**).

STAGING FOR ORAL CANCER

The staging of OCC follows the TNM system and is included in the head and neck chapter of the American Joint Committee on Cancer Staging Manual, eighth edition.[67] OCC and carcinomas from the minor and major salivary glands share the same TNM classification. Oropharyngeal cancers are now stratified using a different TNM system based on the presence or absence of high-risk human papilloma virus and are not discussed in this review.

The TNM system is an algorithm that uses clinical, histologic, and radiological information to stratify the disease. The TNM system helps clinicians to determine the extension of the disease, guide management, standardize clinical trials, and predict prognosis.[67] The T refers to the size and extension of the primary tumor. In OCC, the T category can be assessed through clinical and imaging examination. An important determinant of the T category is the DOI.[67] The DOI is obtained from the initial biopsy or following surgical excision and helps to distinguish exophytic, but less invasive tumors from those ulcerated but more invasive (**Fig. 12, Table 2**).

The N refers to the presence or absence of regional lymphadenopathy. OCC often metastasizes to lymph nodes localized in the neck (40%).[68,69] Cervical lymph nodes can be assessed clinically and radiologically, and the TNM category depends on the number, size, and location of those lymph nodes. The extranodal extension (ENE) refers to the spread of the tumor outside of

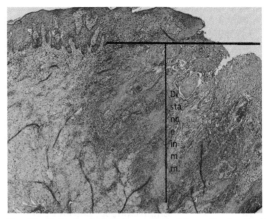

Fig. 12. Pathologic DOI is measured from the level of the basement membrane of the closet adjacent normal mucosa, to the deepest point of tumor invasion. (*Microphotography courtesy of* Dr. Anne C Jones.)

the capsule of the lymph node. ENE is an important modifier of the N category because it greatly affects prognosis.[70] Clinical assessment of ENE is challenging and is recommended to support clinical findings with radiological data to assign an ENE-positive status. Pathologic ENE is determined through histologic examination when histopathology is available (**Table 3**).

The M refers to the presence or absence of distant metastasis and is normally assessed through imaging and laboratory testing. The most common sites of distant metastasis for oral SCC are the lungs, liver, and bones[71] (**Table 4**).[63]

Staging of cancer is a dynamic process that changes as more information is collected during the diagnostic process and treatment. The designation of the prefix "c" is applied when the cancer is being staged based only on clinical features, including imaging (cTNM). The suffix "p" is used when final surgical pathology is available (pTNM) and before adjuvant therapy (radiation or chemotherapy) is initiated.[72]

TREATMENT
Habit Control/Behavioral Modification

Measures to reduce cancer risk factor exposure and promote a healthy lifestyle are recommended to improve overall patient well-being and cancer survivorship. General recommendations include maintaining a healthy weight, following a moderate exercise regimen (eg, ≥150 min/wk of moderate-intensity aerobic exercise), eating a healthy diet, and practicing tobacco cessation and alcohol avoidance.[73]

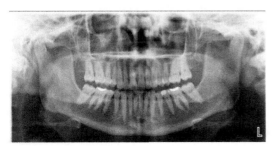

Fig. 11. Panoramic radiograph of a healthy adult. (*Picture courtesy of* Dr. Rujuta Katkar.)

Table 2
T category for oral cavity cancer

T Category	T Criteria
TX	Primary tumor cannot be assessed
Tis	Carcinoma in situ
T1	Tumor ≤2 cm, ≤5 mm DOI
T2	Tumor ≤2 cm, DOI >5 mm and ≤10 mm or tumor >2 cm but ≤4 cm, and ≤10 mm DOI
T3	Tumor >4 cm or any tumor >10 mm DOI
T4	Moderately advanced or very advanced local disease
T4a	Moderately advanced local disease: (lip) tumor invades through cortical bone or involves the inferior alveolar nerve, floor of mouth, or skin of face (ie, chin or nose); (oral cavity) tumor invades adjacent structures only (eg, through cortical bone of the mandible or maxilla, or involves the maxillary sinus or skin of the face); note that superficial erosion of bone/tooth socket (alone) by a gingival primary is not sufficient to classify a tumor as T4
T4b	Very advanced local disease; tumor invades masticator space, pterygoid plates, or skull base and/or encases the internal carotid artery

Adapted from Amin MB, Greene FL, Edge SB, et al. The Eighth Edition AJCC Cancer Staging Manual: Continuing to build a bridge from a population-based to a more "personalized" approach to cancer staging. CA Cancer J Clin 2017;67(2):93-99.

TREATMENT OF ORAL SQUAMOUS CELL CARCINOMA

Surgery and radiotherapy remain the principal treatment options for OSCC.[74,75] The choice of therapy is largely dictated by the TNM staging, which remains the best prognostic predictor for patients with OCC.[67] Detailed stage and site treatment algorithms are available and are continually revised based on the latest clinical trial findings.[75] Of all the oral subsites, the tongue remains the most challenging to predictably treat because of its extensive lymphatic network, lack of anatomic barriers to cancer extension, and propensity for contralateral spread.[76]

Ideally, the therapeutic plan to treat OCC is individualized and developed by a multidisciplinary team (eg, head and neck surgeon, radiation oncologist, medical oncologist, oncology nurse, social worker, speech therapist, nutritionist, dentist, and others). During the treatment planning stage, it is essential that the patient with OCC undergoes a comprehensive medical assessment to identify and address any comorbidities that may impact the planned cancer therapy. Such an approach best aligns communication and care delivery between providers and improves treatment outcomes.[76,77] Efforts to reduce exposure to known risk factors, such as tobacco, heavy alcohol use, and areca nut exposure, should be undertaken.[52]

The patient should also obtain a comprehensive dental evaluation and receive any necessary care to reduce the risk of having to interrupt cancer therapy because of an oral complication. The pretherapy dental evaluation affords the dentist the opportunity to assess the patient's understanding of their disease and their ability to effectively participate in its management. Obtaining necessary dental treatment serves to reduce the risk of potential postcancer therapy complications.[77] Dental extractions should ideally be accomplished at least 2 weeks before radiotherapy is initiated.[77]

Surgery

Whenever feasible, surgical excision remains the therapy of choice to treat OCC.[78] The decision to use surgery is greatly influenced by the tumor location and extent of local invasion.[76] Surgery to manage advanced tumors often results in significant morbidity and the need for the patient to undergo subsequent reconstructive surgery and rehabilitative therapy. Early-stage tumors on the lip, floor of mouth, anterior tongue, and retromolar trigone are highly curable by surgery.[74] Surgical success is predicated on the obtainment of a tumor-free (clear) margin of 5 mm or more.[76] Proper specimen orientation and concise communication between the surgeon and pathologist are essential to ensure accurate margin assessment.[76] Positive (tumor present) margins indicate a need for either re-resection or adjuvant radiotherapy, whereas close margins (ie, <5 mm) should be considered for resection or adjuvant treatment.[78]

All clinically positive necks should undergo a therapeutic neck dissection to determine the extent of ENE and disease burden.[78] The presence of a single metastatic lymph node reduces the 5-year survival rate by half.[78] Because more than 20% of patients with a palpation-negative neck will have an occult neck lymph node, an elective neck dissection should be considered and

Table 3
N category for oral cavity cancer

N Category	N Criteria
NX	Regional lymph nodes cannot be assessed
N0	No regional lymph nodes metastasis
N1	Metastasis in a single ipsilateral lymph node, 3 cm or smaller in greatest dimension and ENE-negative
N2	Metastasis in a single ipsilateral lymph node larger than 3 cm but not larger than 6 cm in greatest dimension and ENE-negative; or metastases in multiple ipsilateral lymph nodes, none larger than 6 cm in greatest dimension and ENE-negative; or metastasis in bilateral or contralateral lymph nodes, none larger than 6 cm in greatest dimension and ENE-negative
N2a	Metastasis in a single ipsilateral lymph node larger than 3 cm but not larger than 6 cm in greatest dimension and ENE-negative
N2b	Metastasis in multiple ipsilateral lymph nodes, none larger than 6 cm in greatest dimension and ENE-negative
N2c	Metastases in bilateral or contralateral lymph nodes, none larger than 6 cm in greatest dimension and ENE-negative
N3	Metastasis in a lymph node larger than 6 cm in greatest dimension and ENE-negative; or metastasis in any lymph nodes and clinically overt ENE-positive
N3a	Metastasis in a lymph node larger than 6 cm in greatest dimension and ENE-negative
N3b	Metastasis in any lymph nodes and clinically overt ENE-positive

Adapted from Amin MB, Greene FL, Edge SB, et al. The Eighth Edition AJCC Cancer Staging Manual: Continuing to build a bridge from a population-based to a more "personalized" approach to cancer staging. CA Cancer J Clin 2017;67(2):93-99.

discussed with the patient during the planning phase.[76]

Radiotherapy

The use of radiotherapy (eg, external beam protocols, brachytherapy, and combinations) as a primary modality to treat OCC is limited by its association with long-term toxicities, such as osteoradionecrosis, hyposalivation, trismus, and others.[76,79] However, radiotherapy may be the best option to accommodate significant functional, cosmetic, or comorbid disease concerns (eg, large lip lesions, anterior tongue lesions, high-risk surgery patients) in the patient with OCC.[79] For locally advanced disease, radiotherapy is often indicated in the adjuvant setting after the initial surgical intervention to improve survival. Contemporary radiotherapy approaches include intensity-modulated radiotherapy and intensity-modulated proton therapy.[76] Both techniques attempt to minimize the adverse outcomes of collateral radiation exposure (eg, dry mouth, muscle fibrosis, trismus, dysphagia).

Chemotherapy

Recent clinical trials demonstrate that chemotherapy is an important adjuvant therapeutic option to manage those patients with advanced disease and/or those with poor prognostic factors, such as ENE, and perineural or lymphatic invasion.[80] It is typically delivered concurrently with radiotherapy, known as chemoradiotherapy, although some patients have benefited from "induction chemotherapy" (**Table 5**).[76]

Chemoradiotherapy has been demonstrated to be superior to radiotherapy alone in treating unresectable OCC and in reducing recurrence of resected tumors in scenarios of positive surgical

Table 4
M category for oral cavity cancer

M Category	M Criteria
MX	Metastasis not determined. Awaiting CT or PET examinations
M0	Distant metastasis not identified
M1	Distant metastasis identified

Adapted from Amin MB, Greene FL, Edge SB, et al. The Eighth Edition AJCC Cancer Staging Manual: Continuing to build a bridge from a population-based to a more "personalized" approach to cancer staging. CA Cancer J Clin 2017;67(2):93-99.

Table 5
Summary of common chemotherapy agents for oral cavity cancer

Indication	Agent
Primary chemoradiotherapy	• Cisplatin • Carboplatin/5-fluorouracil (5-FU) • 5-FU/hydroxyurea • Carboplatin/paclitaxel • Cetuximab • Cisplatin/5-FU • Cisplatin/paclitaxel
Postoperative chemoradiotherapy	• Cisplatin
Induction	• Docetaxel/cisplatin/5-FU • Paclitaxel/cisplatin/5-FU

Data from Hartner L. Chemotherapy for Oral Cancer. Dent Clin North Am 2018;62(1):87-97.

margins and ENE. The chemotherapy agent acts a radiation sensitizer to reduce the development of radiation resistance.[76] Current consensus guidelines recommend the use of primary or adjuvant chemoradiation be determined on a case-by-case basis for patients at high risk for recurrence.[69] Cisplatin is the first-line agent of choice, although it is associated with significant adverse effects to include renal failure, myelosuppression, ototoxicity, neuropathy, nausea, and vomiting.[75,80] The alternative drug carboplatin is associated with a greater risk of myelosuppression than cisplatin, but avoids the cisplatin-related risks of nephropathy, ototoxicity, and neuropathy.[80] The use of induction chemotherapy before initial primary treatment remains unclear, and further research is necessary.

Targeted Agents and Immunotherapy

Numerous chemotherapy regimens to treat unresponsive or metastatic OCC are available to consider, but specific validated protocols remain to be established. The regimen of the antimetabolite gemcitabine plus the antimicrotubular paclitaxel or the regimen of paclitaxel plus the EGFR inhibitor cetuximab may be used as initial therapy for patients unable to tolerate platinum-based therapies.[80] Two PD-1 monoclonal antibodies, nivolumab and pembrolizumab, are approved by the Food and Drug Administration

to treat metastatic disease with progression on or after platinum-based therapy.[76,80] All of these therapies incur some level of adverse risk, and when choosing therapy, the prior treatment history and the patient's ability and desire to tolerate the chosen therapy must be considered.

TREATMENT OF ORAL POTENTIALLY MALIGNANT DISORDERS

In contrast to the treatment of OCC, there are no evidence-based treatments for OPMDs. All patients should be counseled on the importance of reducing predisposing risk factors, such as tobacco, alcohol exposure, and areca nut exposure.[81] Validated chemoprevention regimens (eg, antioxidants, retinoids, cyclooxygenase inhibitors, epidermal growth factor inhibitors) remain elusive.[82]

Because the malignant transformation rate of OPMDs is approximately 1.36% per year,[14] the challenge is to triage those lesions at highest risk. For a given OPMD, a specific management protocol is typically based on a careful clinical and histopathologic risk assessment of the lesion at hand. Factors associated with increased risk of malignant transformation include female gender, non-smoking status, age greater than 45 years, nonhomogeneous leukoplakia, high-grade dysplasia, size greater than200 mm^2, and high-risk subsite.[52]

OPMDs demonstrating high-grade OED should ideally be excised. Available methodologies include scalpel excision, laser excision/ablation, cryotherapy, and photodynamic therapy.[52] All patients who undergo excision/ablation must undergo lifelong monitoring for OPMD recurrence or development of a new OPMD.[82] There are no validated standardized protocols addressing the frequency of such monitoring, but reassessment every 3 to 6 months has been suggested.[82] High-risk lesions for which excision or ablation is not a viable option (ie, large size, multifocal disease, or medical contraindications) should be carefully reassessed for disease evolution as described above.

In a similar fashion, low-risk OPMDs are recommended to be reassessed for change at a frequency of every 6 to 12 months.

SUMMARY

Not all patients with OCC or OPMDs seek care from a dentist. It is therefore essential that health care providers, such as dermatologists, appreciate and recognize the risk factors and signs and symptoms of OCC and OPMDs, because early detection is critical to improving outcomes. Patients suspected of having either OCC or an OPMD should be referred to an oral health care provider for appropriate evaluation and management.

The heterogeneous genetic and epigenetic landscape of OCC has complicated the application of precision therapeutic strategies to manage OCC. Putative candidate biomarkers that may be useful in the future to improve the diagnosis, prognosis, and management have yet to be validated. Until such validation is established, the conventional visual and tactile oral cavity examination followed by biopsy and histologic analysis of OPMDs remains the gold standard to establish a definitive diagnosis. Patients diagnosed with OSCC should be referred to and managed by a multidisciplinary team. Because of the variable malignant transformation rate, patients with an OPMD, irrespective of whether they are diagnosed with OED, should be closely monitored. Demographic, clinical, and histologic parameters, such as patient gender, age, habits, location, and size of the OPMD and degree of OED, collectively contribute to risk for malignant transformation. In general, measures to reduce modifiable cancer risk factor exposures and promotion of a healthy lifestyle are recommended and should be reinforced by all health care providers to improve overall patient well-being and cancer survivorship.

REFERENCES

1. Siegel RL, Miller KD, Jemal A. Cancer statistics, 2019. CA Cancer J Clin 2019;69(1):7–34.
2. Gillison ML, Koch WM, Capone RB, et al. Evidence for a causal association between human papillomavirus and a subset of head and neck cancers. J Natl Cancer Inst 2000;92(9):709–20.
3. Joseph AW, D'Souza G. Epidemiology of human papillomavirus-related head and neck cancer. Otolaryngol Clin North Am 2012;45(4):739–64.
4. Vidal L, Gillison ML. Human papillomavirus in HNSCC: recognition of a distinct disease type. Hematol Oncol Clin North Am 2008;22(6):1125–42, vii.
5. Warnakulasuriya S, Johnson NW, van der Waal I. Nomenclature and classification of potentially malignant disorders of the oral mucosa. J Oral Pathol Med 2007;36(10):575–80.
6. Howlader N, Noone AM, Krapcho M, et al. SEER cancer statistics review, 1975-2016. Bethesda (MD): National Cancer Institute; 2019.
7. Van Dyne EA, Henley SJ, Saraiya M, et al. Trends in human papillomavirus-associated cancers - United States, 1999-2015. MMWR Morb Mortal Wkly Rep 2018;67(33):918–24.
8. Van der Waal I. Potentially malignant disorders of the oral and oropharyngeal mucosa; terminology, classification and present concepts of management. Oral Oncol 2009;45(4–5):317–23.
9. Mawardi H, Elad S, Correa ME, et al. Oral epithelial dysplasia and squamous cell carcinoma following allogeneic hematopoietic stem cell transplantation: clinical presentation and treatment outcomes. Bone Marrow Transplant 2011; 46(6):884–91.
10. McBride KA, Ballinger ML, Killick E, et al. Li-Fraumeni syndrome: cancer risk assessment and clinical management. Nat Rev Clin Oncol 2014;11(5): 260–71.
11. Scully C, Langdon J, Evans J. Marathon of eponyms: 26 Zinsser-Engman-Cole syndrome (dyskeratosis congenita). Oral Dis 2012;18(5):522–3.
12. Furquim CP, Pivovar A, Amenabar JM, et al. Oral cancer in Fanconi anemia: review of 121 cases. Crit Rev Oncol Hematol 2018;125:35–40.
13. Mello FW, Miguel AFP, Dutra KL, et al. Prevalence of oral potentially malignant disorders: a systematic review and meta-analysis. J Oral Pathol Med 2018; 47(7):633–40.
14. Petti S. Pooled estimate of world leukoplakia prevalence: a systematic review. Oral Oncol 2003;39(8): 770–80.
15. van der Waal I. Oral potentially malignant disorders: is malignant transformation predictable and preventable? Med Oral Patol Oral Cir Bucal 2014;19(4): e386–90.
16. Reichart PA, Philipsen HP. Oral erythroplakia–a review. Oral Oncol 2005;41(6):551–61.
17. Bouquot JE, Ephros H. Erythroplakia: the dangerous red mucosa. Pract Periodontics Aesthet Dent 1995; 7(6):59–67 [quiz: 68].
18. Speight PM, Khurram SA, Kujan O. Oral potentially malignant disorders: risk of progression to malignancy. Oral Surg Oral Med Oral Pathol Oral Radiol 2018;125(6):612–27.
19. Iocca O, Sollecito TP, Alawi F, et al. Potentially malignant disorders of the oral cavity and oral dysplasia: a systematic review and meta-analysis of malignant transformation rate by subtype. Head Neck 2020; 42(3):539–55.
20. Villa A, Hanna GJ, Kacew A, et al. Oral keratosis of unknown significance shares genomic overlap with oral dysplasia. Oral Dis 2019;25(7):1707–14.
21. Holmstrup P, Vedtofte P, Reibel J, et al. Long-term treatment outcome of oral premalignant lesions. Oral Oncol 2006;42(5):461–74.
22. Gonzalez-Moles MA, Ruiz-Avila I, Gonzalez-Ruiz L, et al. Malignant transformation risk of oral lichen planus: a systematic review and comprehensive meta-analysis. Oral Oncol 2019;96:121–30.
23. Murti PR, Bhonsle RB, Pindborg JJ, et al. Malignant transformation rate in oral submucous fibrosis over a 17-year period. Community Dent Oral Epidemiol 1985;13(6):340–1.
24. Arakeri G, Patil SG, Aljabab AS, et al. Oral submucous fibrosis: an update on pathophysiology of

malignant transformation. J Oral Pathol Med 2017; 46(6):413–7.

25. Hansen LS, Olson JA, Silverman S Jr. Proliferative verrucous leukoplakia. A long-term study of thirty patients. Oral Surg Oral Med Oral Pathol 1985; 60(3):285–98.

26. Bagan JV, Jimenez-Soriano Y, Diaz-Fernandez JM, et al. Malignant transformation of proliferative verrucous leukoplakia to oral squamous cell carcinoma: a series of 55 cases. Oral Oncol 2011;47(8):732–5.

27. Lopes MLDdS, Silva Júnior FLd, Lima KC, et al. Clinicopathological profile and management of 161 cases of actinic cheilitis. An Bras Dermatol 2015; 90(4):505–12.

28. Pimentel NDR, Michalany N, Alchorne M, et al. Actinic cheilitis: histopathology and p53. J Cutan Pathol 2006;33(8):539–44.

29. Gomes JO, de Vasconcelos Carvalho M, Fonseca FP, et al. CD1a+ and CD83+ Langerhans cells are reduced in lower lip squamous cell carcinoma. J Oral Pathol Med 2016;45(6):433–9.

30. IARC Working Group on the Evaluation of Carcinogenic Risks to Humans. Tobacco Smoke and Involuntary Smoking. Lyon (FR): International Agency for Research on Cancer; 2004. (IARC Monographs on the Evaluation of Carcinogenic Risks to Humans, No. 83.) Available at: https://www.ncbi.nlm.nih.gov/books/NBK316407/.

31. IARC Working Group on the Evaluation of Carcinogenic Risk to Humans. Smokeless Tobacco and Some Tobacco-specific N-Nitrosamines. Lyon (FR): International Agency for Research on Cancer; 2007. (IARC Monographs on the Evaluation of Carcinogenic Risks to Humans, No. 89.) Available at: https://www.ncbi.nlm.nih.gov/books/NBK326497/.

32. IARC Working Group on the Evaluation of Carcinogenic Risk to Humans. Personal Habits and Indoor Combustions. Lyon (FR): International Agency for Research on Cancer; 2012. (IARC Monographs on the Evaluation of Carcinogenic Risks to Humans, No. 100E.) Available at: https://www.ncbi.nlm.nih.gov/books/NBK304391/.

33. IARC Working Group on the Evaluation of Carcinogenic Risk to Humans. Betel-quid and Areca-nut Chewing and Some Areca-nut-derived Nitrosamines. Lyon (FR): International Agency for Research on Cancer; 2004. (IARC Monographs on the Evaluation of Carcinogenic Risks to Humans, No. 85.) Available at: https://www.ncbi.nlm.nih.gov/books/NBK316567/.

34. Conway DI, Brenner DR, McMahon AD, et al. Estimating and explaining the effect of education and income on head and neck cancer risk: INHANCE consortium pooled analysis of 31 case-control studies from 27 countries. Int J Cancer 2015;136(5):1125–39.

35. Chuang SC, Jenab M, Heck JE, et al. Diet and the risk of head and neck cancer: a pooled analysis in the INHANCE consortium. Cancer Causes Control 2012;23(1):69–88.

36. Hashim D, Sartori S, Brennan P, et al. The role of oral hygiene in head and neck cancer: results from International Head and Neck Cancer Epidemiology (INHANCE) consortium. Ann Oncol 2016;27(8): 1619–25.

37. Javed F, Warnakulasuriya S. Is there a relationship between periodontal disease and oral cancer? A systematic review of currently available evidence. Crit Rev Oncol Hematol 2016;97:197–205.

38. Dietrich T, Reichart PA, Scheifele C. Clinical risk factors of oral leukoplakia in a representative sample of the US population. Oral Oncol 2004;40(2): 158–63.

39. Morse DE, Psoter WJ, Cleveland D, et al. Smoking and drinking in relation to oral cancer and oral epithelial dysplasia. Cancer Causes Control 2007; 18(9):919–29.

40. Li CC, Shen Z, Bavarian R, et al. Oral cancer: genetics and the role of precision medicine. Surg Oncol Clin N Am 2020;29(1):127–44.

41. Braakhuis BJ, Tabor MP, Kummer JA, et al. A genetic explanation of Slaughter's concept of field cancerization: evidence and clinical implications. Cancer Res 2003;63(8):1727–30.

42. Mehanna HM, Rattay T, Smith J, et al. Treatment and follow-up of oral dysplasia - a systematic review and meta-analysis. Head Neck 2009;31(12):1600–9.

43. Zhang L, Poh CF, Williams M, et al. Loss of heterozygosity (LOH) profiles–validated risk predictors for progression to oral cancer. Cancer Prev Res (Phila) 2012;5(9):1081–9.

44. Warnakulasuriya S, Ariyawardana A. Malignant transformation of oral leukoplakia: a systematic review of observational studies. J Oral Pathol Med 2016;45(3):155–66.

45. Sankaranarayanan R. Screening for cancer in low- and middle-income countries. Ann Glob Health 2014;80(5):412–7.

46. Rajaraman P, Anderson BO, Basu P, et al. Recommendations for screening and early detection of common cancers in India. Lancet Oncol 2015; 16(7):e352–61.

47. Speight PM, Epstein J, Kujan O, et al. Screening for oral cancer-a perspective from the Global Oral Cancer Forum. Oral Surg Oral Med Oral Pathol Oral Radiol 2017;123(6):680–7.

48. Moyer VA. Screening for oral cancer: U.S. Preventive Services Task Force recommendation statement. Ann Intern Med 2014;160(1):55–60.

49. AAOM Clinical Practice Statement: subject: oral cancer examination and screening. Oral Surg Oral Med Oral Pathol Oral Radiol 2016;122(2):174–5.

50. Lingen MW, Abt E, Agrawal N, et al. Evidence-based clinical practice guideline for the evaluation of potentially malignant disorders in the oral cavity: a

report of the American Dental Association. J Am Dent Assoc 2017;148(10):712–27.e10.

51. Sollecito TP, Stoopler ET. Clinical approaches to oral mucosal disorders: part II. Preface. Dent Clin North Am 2014;58(2):xi–xii.

52. Nadeau C, Kerr AR. Evaluation and management of oral potentially malignant disorders. Dent Clin North Am 2018;62(1):1–27.

53. Lam DK, Schmidt BL. Orofacial pain onset predicts transition to head and neck cancer. Pain 2011; 152(5):1206–9.

54. Rhodus NL, Kerr AR, Patel K. Oral cancer: leukoplakia, premalignancy, and squamous cell carcinoma. Dent Clin North Am 2014;58(2):315–40.

55. Rhodus NL. Oral cancer update: 2017. Northwest Dent 2017;96(1):21–3, 25–7.

56. Napier SS, Speight PM. Natural history of potentially malignant oral lesions and conditions: an overview of the literature. J Oral Pathol Med 2008;37(1):1–10.

57. Villa A, Menon RS, Kerr AR, et al. Proliferative leukoplakia: proposed new clinical diagnostic criteria. Oral Dis 2018;24(5):749–60.

58. Rao NR, Villa A, More CB, et al. Oral submucous fibrosis: a contemporary narrative review with a proposed inter-professional approach for an early diagnosis and clinical management. J Otolaryngol Head Neck Surg 2020;49(1):3.

59. Salgueiro AP, de Jesus LH, de Souza IF, et al. Treatment of actinic cheilitis: a systematic review. Clin Oral Investig 2019;23(5):2041–53.

60. Huber MA. Adjunctive diagnostic techniques for oral and oropharyngeal cancer discovery. Dent Clin North Am 2018;62(1):59–75.

61. Lingen MW, Tampi MP, Urquhart O, et al. Adjuncts for the evaluation of potentially malignant disorders in the oral cavity: diagnostic test accuracy systematic review and meta-analysis-a report of the American Dental Association. J Am Dent Assoc 2017; 148(11):797–813 e52.

62. Siriwardena S, Tsunematsu T, Qi G, et al. Invasion-related factors as potential diagnostic and therapeutic targets in oral squamous cell carcinoma-a review. Int J Mol Sci 2018;19(5).

63. Neville BW, Damm DD, Allen CM, et al. Epithelial pathology. In: Oral and maxillofacial pathology. Elsevier Health Sciences; 2015.

64. Wong RJ, Keel SB, Glynn RJ, et al. Histological pattern of mandibular invasion by oral squamous cell carcinoma. Laryngoscope 2000;110(1):65–72.

65. Cracchiolo JR, Xu B, Migliacci JC, et al. Patterns of recurrence in oral tongue cancer with perineural invasion. Head Neck 2018;40(6):1287–95.

66. Mupparapu M, Shanti RM. Evaluation and staging of oral cancer. Dent Clin North Am 2018;62(1):47–58.

67. Lydiatt WM, Patel SG, O'Sullivan B, et al. Head and neck cancers-major changes in the American Joint Committee on Cancer Eighth Edition Cancer Staging Manual. CA Cancer J Clin 2017;67(2):122–37.

68. Okura M, Aikawa T, Sawai NY, et al. Decision analysis and treatment threshold in a management for the N0 neck of the oral cavity carcinoma. Oral Oncol 2009;45(10):908–11.

69. Noguti J, De Moura CF, De Jesus GP, et al. Metastasis from oral cancer: an overview. Cancer Genomics Proteomics 2012;9(5):329–35.

70. Wreesmann VB, Katabi N, Palmer FL, et al. Influence of extracapsular nodal spread extent on prognosis of oral squamous cell carcinoma. Head Neck 2016;38(Suppl 1):E1192–9.

71. Sumioka S, Sawai NY, Kishino M, et al. Risk factors for distant metastasis in squamous cell carcinoma of the oral cavity. J Oral Maxillofac Surg 2013; 71(7):1291–7.

72. Amin MB, Greene FL, Edge SB, et al. The Eighth Edition AJCC Cancer Staging Manual: continuing to build a bridge from a population-based to a more "personalized" approach to cancer staging. CA Cancer J Clin 2017;67(2):93–9.

73. Ligibel J. Lifestyle factors in cancer survivorship. J Clin Oncol 2012;30(30):3697–704.

74. National Cancer Institute lip and oral cavity cancer treatment (PDQ®) - health professional version. National Cancer Institute. Available at: https://www.cancer.gov/types/head-and-neck/hp/adult/lip-mouth-treatment-pdq. Accessed November 11, 2019.

75. National Comprehensive Cancer Network: NCCN Practice Guidelines in Oncology: head and neck cancers. 2019. Available at: https://www.nccn.org/professionals/physician_gls/pdf/head-and-neck.pdf. Accessed November 11, 2019.

76. Chinn SB, Myers JN. Oral cavity carcinoma: current management, controversies, and future directions. J Clin Oncol 2015;33(29):3269–76.

77. Levi LE, Lalla RV. Dental treatment planning for the patient with oral cancer. Dent Clin North Am 2018; 62(1):121–30.

78. Shanti RM, O'Malley BW Jr. Surgical management of oral cancer. Dent Clin North Am 2018;62(1):77–86.

79. Lin A. Radiation therapy for oral cavity and oropharyngeal cancers. Dent Clin North Am 2018;62(1): 99–109.

80. Hartner L. Chemotherapy for oral cancer. Dent Clin North Am 2018;62(1):87–97.

81. Vladimirov BS, Schiodt M. The effect of quitting smoking on the risk of unfavorable events after surgical treatment of oral potentially malignant lesions. Int J Oral Maxillofac Surg 2009;38(11):1188–93.

82. Awadallah M, Idle M, Patel K, et al. Management update of potentially premalignant oral epithelial lesions. Oral Surg Oral Med Oral Pathol Oral Radiol 2018;125(6):628–36.

Adverse Drug Events in the Oral Cavity

Anna Yuan, DMD, PhD[a],*, Sook-Bin Woo, DMD, MMSc[b,c]

KEYWORDS

- Adverse drug events • Drug-related side effects • Adverse reactions • Medications • Oral cavity
- Targeted therapies

KEY POINTS

- Adverse drug events in the oral cavity are common and will likely increase as newer therapeutic agents are approved.
- This review describes common and uncommon oral mucosal reactions to medications, namely hyposalivation, ulcerative and red and white mucosal lesions, pigmentation, fibrovascular hyperplasia, reactive keratosis, dysesthesia, osteonecrosis, infection, angioedema, and malignancy.
- Health care providers should be familiar with such events in their practice.

INTRODUCTION

Most medications have the potential of eliciting an adverse reaction from patients. "Adverse drug reaction" was defined by Edwards and Aronson[1] in 2000 as "an appreciably harmful or unpleasant reaction, resulting from an intervention related to the use of a medicinal product, which predicts hazard from future administration and warrants prevention or specific treatment, or alteration of the dosage regimen, or withdrawal of the product." This definition excludes minor reactions, addresses the issue of medication error, addresses injury from nonpharmaceutical agents (including contaminants and inactive ingredients), and does not assign disease mechanism. The current term that satisfies regulatory bodies and patient safety advocates is "adverse drug event" (ADE), which includes (1) harm caused by a drug (commonly known as adverse drug reaction), (2) harm caused by appropriate drug use (usually referred to as a side effect), and (3) medication errors.[2] This review focuses on the clinical presentations of the common ADEs as defined by Nebeker and colleagues.[2]

Typically, an ADE is detected within hours, days, or months after taking the medications depending on the specific type of reaction. Lichenoid drug reactions may present asymptomatically initially (reticular/keratotic lesions) and can become symptomatic years later (when ulcerated or erythematous), making the relationship between onset of drug use and development of ADE difficult to ascertain. The presence of the oral condition predating the administration of the medication must be excluded and this may be difficult to determine if the patient has not been evaluated by a health care provider on a regular basis. Resolution should occur after discontinuation of the suspected medication, although this may necessitate the use of topical corticosteroids for management of inflammatory conditions. Recurrence with rechallenge confirms the diagnosis, although this may not be feasible if the ADEs are unpleasant, severe, or life-threatening. Concurrent medications must be noted.

Drug-induced cutaneous reactions are common and varied in presentation, but only a limited number of reaction patterns occur in the oral cavity.

[a] Division of Oral Medicine, Tufts University School of Dental Medicine, 1 Kneeland Street, Boston, MA 02111, USA; [b] Division of Oral Medicine and Dentistry, Brigham and Women's Hospital, 75 Francis Street, Boston, MA 02115, USA; [c] Department of Oral Medicine, Infection and Immunity, Harvard School of Dental Medicine, 188 Longwood Avenue, Boston, MA 02115, USA
* Corresponding author.
E-mail address: anna.yuan@tufts.edu

Dermatol Clin 38 (2020) 523–533
https://doi.org/10.1016/j.det.2020.05.012
0733-8635/20/© 2020 Elsevier Inc. All rights reserved.

This is likely caused by the higher turnover rate in the oral mucosa compared with the skin, which does not allow for the spectrum of clinical changes detectable on the skin. The oral lesions to be discussed fall into several categories (**Box 1**).

HYPOSALIVATION/XEROSTOMIA

Medication use is one of the most common causes of xerostomia and hyposalivation, and more than 80% of the 100 most prescribed medications in the United States may result in this effect, including new targeted therapies (**Box 2**).[3,4] Many middle aged and older patients in the United States are on multiple medications (polypharmacy), and even medications with a small anticholinergic effect may act synergistically when used in combination to cause oral symptoms of dryness and discomfort (**Fig. 1**).

LICHENOID REACTION/LICHEN PLANUS

Many medications are known to cause cutaneous lichenoid hypersensitivity reactions (LHR), which are often difficult to distinguish clinically and histopathologically from idiopathic cutaneous lichen planus (LP).[5] It has been postulated that active thiol groups found in the chemical structure of medications, such as piroxicam, sulfasalazine, and glipizide, play a role in inciting such reactions (**Box 3**).[6] It is likely, therefore, that these same medications may cause oral LHR; idiopathic and medication-induced oral LP/LHR are indistinguishable. Thyroid disease (eg, hypothyroidism and Hashimoto thyroiditis) and/or treatment with levothyroxine are also strongly associated with the development of LP/LHR (**Fig. 2**).[5,7]

The two classes of medications historically associated with oral LHR are nonsteroidal anti-inflammatory drugs (NSAIDs) and antihypertensive agents including β-blockers, angiotensin-converting enzyme (ACE) inhibitors, and diuretics (in particular hydrochlorothiazide).[8] Sulfonylurea antidiabetic medications (eg, tolbutamide, glipizide, and glimepiride), antifungals (eg, ketoconazole), anticonvulsants (eg, carbamazepine), immunomodulatory drugs (eg, gold salts and penicillamine), sulfasalazine, allopurinol, and lithium have been reported to elicit oral LHRs.[9] More recently, anti–programmed death receptor-1 (PD-1) immunotherapies, such as nivolumab and pembrolizumab, have been associated with oral LHRs, or with nonspecific red and/or white changes (**Fig. 3**).[10,11] This may be caused by epithelial cell apoptosis and basement membrane alterations caused by inhibition of the PD-1 ligand pathway.[10]

Box 1
Drug-induced oral reactions

Hyposalivation/xerostomia

Lichenoid reaction/lichen planus

Aphthous-like and nonaphthous-like ulcers

Bullous disorders

Pigmentation

Fibrovascular hyperplasia

Reactive keratosis/epithelial hyperplasia

Dysesthesias

Osteonecrosis of the jaws

Infection

Angioedema

Malignancy and leukoplakia

Box 2
Medication classes associated with hyposalivation

Antidepressants

Antipsychotics

Antihistamines

Muscarinic receptor

α-Receptor antagonists

Antihypertensives (diuretics, β-blockers, angiotensin-converting enzyme inhibitors)

Bronchodilators

Skeletal muscle relaxants

Chemotherapy agents

Appetite suppressants

Decongestants

Antimigraine drugs

Opioids

Benzodiazepines

Hypnotics

H_2 receptor antagonists and proton-pump inhibitors

Systemic retinoids

Anti–human immunodeficiency virus medications

Cytokine therapy

Targeted therapies (lenvatinib, sunitinib, bevacizumab, nivolumab, dacomitinib)

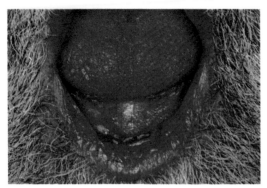

Fig. 1. Hyposalivation from polypharmacy: desiccated, shiny tongue, floor of mouth, and lips with no floor of mouth pooling and foamy saliva.

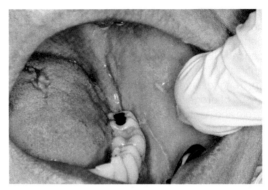

Fig. 2. Hypothyroidism and levothyroxine-associated lichenoid reaction: note typical striations on the left buccal mucosa.

HMG-CoA inhibitors, such as pravastatin, simvastatin, fluvastatin, and lovastatin, have been implicated in causing cutaneous LHR with mucosal involvement,[12] as have other medications, such as imatinib and letrozole.[13,14] Asarch and colleagues[15] reported two cases of oral LP (more accurately LHR) in patients taking tumor necrosis factor (TNF)-α inhibitors infliximab and adalimumab, and 12 cases involving TNF receptor fusion proteins etanercept and abatacept. Infliximab and certolizumab used to treat Crohn disease have been linked to biopsy-proven oral LP.[16,17] This seems paradoxic because oral LP is mediated by TNF-α. However, it has been suggested that when TNF-α is inhibited, there may be upregulation of interferon-α,[15] which then activates T cells and dendritic cells, causing an inflammatory response.[18] The novel anti-CD20 monoclonal antibody obinutuzumab was reported to cause LHR on the skin and oral ulcers.[19]

Fixed drug eruptions (FDEs) in the oral cavity are uncommon and recur at the same site and range from bullous, erosive, hyperpigmented, pruritic, or erythematous lesions each time the offending medication is ingested, and there may be skin or

---

Box 3
Medication classes associated with lichenoid hypersensitivity reactions

Levothyroxine

Nonsteroidal anti-inflammatory drugs (piroxicam)

Antihypertensives (diuretics in particular hydrochlorothiazide, β-blockers, angiotensin-converting enzyme inhibitors)

Sulfonylurea antidiabetics (tolbutamide, glipizide, glimepiride)

Antifungals (ketoconazole)

Anticonvulsants (carbamazepine)

Immunomodulatory drugs (gold salts, penicillamine)

Sulfasalazine

Allopurinol

Lithium

Anti–programmed death receptor-1 immunotherapies (nivolumab, pembrolizumab)

HMG-CoA inhibitors (pravastatin, simvastatin, fluvastatin, lovastatin)

Imatinib

Aromatase inhibitors (letrozole)

Anti–tumor necrosis factor-α monoclonal antibodies (infliximab, adalimumab, certolizumab)

Tumor necrosis factor-α receptor fusion proteins (etanercept, abatacept)

Anti-CD20 monoclonal antibodies (obinutuzumab)

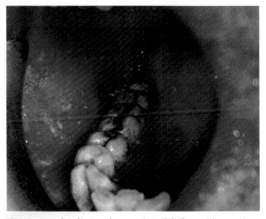

Fig. 3. Pembrolizumab-associated lichenoid reaction: erythema and papular keratosis but with slight striations.

genital involvement; oral involvement alone was noted in 14.8% of patients.[20] First- and second-generation antihistamines have been known to cause FDEs on the skin, and the third-generation antihistamine levocetirizine caused FDE of the lip, tongue, and glans penis.[21,22] Almost half of cases of orogenital FDEs are caused by cotrimoxazole and naproxen with cotrimoxazole causing lesions on the tongue,[20] whereas fluconazole was linked to erosive lesions of the palatal mucosa and oral bullae.[23,24] Tetracycline, clarithromycin, tinidazole, oxyphenbutazone, gabapentin, simvastatin, and silodosin have also been associated with oral FDEs.[25–29]

APHTHOUS-LIKE AND NONAPHTHOUS-LIKE ULCERS

NSAIDs were one of the earliest classes of drugs associated with the development of aphthous-like ulcers in the oral cavity. Piroxicam in particular was demonstrated to cause such ulcers possibly because it contains a thiol group.[30] Naproxen, trimethoprim-sulfamethoxazole, cyclooxygenase-2 inhibitors (eg, refecoxib), and the angiotensin receptor blocker losartan have been implicated in the development of aphthous-like ulcers.[31,32]

Aphthous-like ulcers (reported as mucositis) have been documented in up to 70% of patients with metastatic tumors treated with mechanistic target of rapamycin inhibitors including sirolimus, temsirolimus, everolimus, and ridaforolimus (Fig. 4).[33,34] However, unlike patients with idiopathic recurrent aphthous ulcers, these regress completely on withdrawal of therapy without recurrence.

Conventional chemotherapy agents, such as 5-fluorouracil, cisplatin, methotrexate, and hydroxyurea, are stomatoxic and cause oral ulcers and ulcerative mucositis (Fig. 5).[35] These ulcers tend to be larger and more diffuse and do not have the ovoid, well-demarcated appearance of aphthous ulcers. Mycophenolate mofetil and tacrolimus have been reported to cause ulcers on the tongue, palatal mucosa, labial mucosa, and gingiva in solid organ transplant patients that resolve with cessation of medication.[36] Rare cases of ulcers associated with multitargeted kinase inhibitors (MTKIs) exist.[37]

BULLOUS DISORDERS

Medication-induced autoimmune bullous disorders of the skin are not uncommon, whereas such disorders presenting in the oral cavity are rare.[38] The development of simultaneous oral and cutaneous pemphigus vulgaris has been

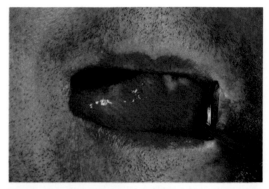

Fig. 4. Everolimus-induced aphthous-like ulcer: note three pseudomembranous ulcers on the lateral, ventral, and tip of tongue.

noted with thiol radical-containing drugs, such as penicillamine, and NSAIDs.[39,40] Cutaneous bullous pemphigoid has been associated with antipsychotic medications, spironolactones, sulfonamides, antihypertensives, and oral hypoglycemic agents.[41,42] Patients on checkpoint inhibitors, such as nivolumab, ipilimumab, and durvalumab, may develop oral and skin involvement by bullous pemphigoid.[43] The clinical course of checkpoint inhibitor–induced bullous pemphigoid differs in that it may persist long after the discontinuation of the offending medication, possibly because of the continued in vivo effect of immune checkpoint inhibition and subsequent continued immune activation.[43] Erythema multiforme of the skin and oral mucous membranes has been reported with the administration of infliximab and adalimumab,[44,45] and in the oral cavity with cotrimoxazole.[46]

Stevens-Johnson syndrome and toxic epidermal necrolysis are severe necrolytic hypersensitivity reactions that, unlike erythema multiforme, are much more commonly associated with the use of medications and may be life-

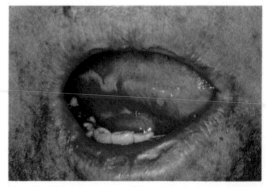

Fig. 5. Ulcerative mucositis secondary to chemotherapy: note small ulcer and larger diffuse ulcer on the right lateral ventral tongue.

threatening.[47] Allopurinol, antimicrobials (eg, amoxicillin/clavulanic acid), anticonvulsants, and most recently PD-1 inhibitors (eg, pembrolizumab) have been implicated.[48,49] In Han Chinese populations, Stevens-Johnson syndrome and toxic epidermal necrolysis caused by anticonvulsants, such as phenobarbital, phenytoin, and carbamazepine, are associated with HLA-B*1502, whereas reactions to allopurinol are associated with HLA-B*5801 universally.[50,51] Many HLA-types are associated with drug hypersensitivity reactions and it may be that in the future, pharmacogenomic screening may become the norm before prescription of such medications.[52]

PIGMENTATION

Metabolites of medications, such as the tetracyclines, minocyclines, antimalarial drugs (hydroxychloroquine, mepacrine, and quinacrine), and phenazine dyes (clofazimine), may deposit in the oral mucosa. Such drug metabolites chelate with iron and melanin resulting in pigmentation of the hard palatal mucosa, which have specific histopathology.[53] Tetracycline and minocycline also deposit in the teeth, bones, thyroid, and sclera, and cause mucosal and nail pigmentation.[54] The tyrosine kinase inhibitor imatinib can cause hyperpigmentation or hypopigmentation of skin, hyperpigmentation of nails, and diffuse blue-grey pigmentation on the palatal mucosa with similar characteristic histopathology (**Fig. 6**).[55]

Other medications that have been noted to cause oral mucosal pigmentation are zidovudine; oral contraceptives; and chemotherapy agents, such as doxorubicin, docetaxel, and cyclophosphamide.[56] Pigmentation of the facial skin has been noted with the use of amiodorone and phenothiazines (chlorpromazine).[57,58]

FIBROVASCULAR HYPERPLASIA

Calcium channel blockers, in particular nifedipine and amlodipine, are antihypertensive agents that often induce hyperplasia of the gingival tissues.[59] It has been suggested that the mechanism is caused by decreased cellular folic acid uptake leading to decreased activity of matrix metalloproteinases and the failure to activate collagenase. As such, folate supplementation may mitigate this effect.[60]

Calcineurin inhibitors, such as cyclosporine, or less frequently, tacrolimus, also induce localized polyploid fibrovascular tumors often on the tongue and buccal mucosa rather than gingiva (**Fig. 7**).[61] The increased production of collagen is thought to be caused by the reduced activity of matrix metalloproteinases and the increased activity of tissue

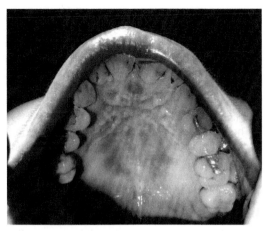

Fig. 6. Pigmentation associated with imatinib: diffuse blue-gray macule of the palatal mucosa.

inhibitors of metalloproteinases.[62] It has also been proposed that phenytoin and cyclosporine A increase expression of interleukin-1 and -6, which may induce oral mucosal mesenchymal stem cells to differentiate toward a profibrotic phenotype.[63]

REACTIVE KERATOSIS/EPITHELIAL HYPERPLASIA

Palifermin is a recombinant keratinocyte growth factor that reduces the incidence and severity of mucositis related to autologous hematopoietic stem cell transplantation and cytoreductive therapy.[64,65] It has been associated with diffuse, thickened white plaques in the mouth in approximately 18% of cases.[66,67] BRAF inhibitors have been reported to cause BRAF-inhibitor-associated verrucous keratoses of the skin.[68]

DYSESTHESIAS

Oral dysesthesias, such as sensitivity, burning, dysgeusia, and other altered sensations without

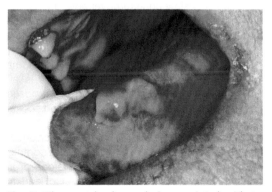

Fig. 7. Fibrovascular hyperplasia associated with tacrolimus: ulcerated nodule on the left lateral tongue.

clinical signs, may be caused by medications. A study on the prevalence of dysgeusia and dysosmia was reported for several drug classes including macrolides, such as clarithromycin (17%),[69] antimycotics, such as terbinafine (9%), fluoroquinolones (8%), and kinase inhibitors, ACE-inhibitors, statins, and proton-pump inhibitors (3%–5% each).[70]

The mechanism is multifactorial, and may be a combination of drug-receptor inhibition; alteration of neurotransmitter function; disturbance of action potentials in neurons; and dysfunctional sensory modulation in the brain attributed to neuronopathy, axonopathy, myelinopathy, and intraepidermal nerve fiber degeneration.[71] Chemotherapy-associated peripheral neuropathies are often associated with the use of taxanes; platinum compounds; thalidomide; bortezomib; and vinca alkaloids, such as vincristine and vinblastine.[69,72]

The development of oral dysesthesias is significantly associated with the development and severity of palmar-plantar erythrodysesthesia in patients on MTKIs.[73] Stomatitis symptoms have been reported in 26% of patients on sorafenib and 36% to 60% of patients on sunitinib in the absence of oral findings.[74] The anaplastic lymphoma kinase inhibitor crizotinib, tyrosine kinase inhibitor pazopanib, mechanistic target of rapamycin inhibitor everolimus, and human epidermal growth factor receptor (EGFR/HER-1) tyrosine kinase inhibitors dacomitinib and afatinib have also been linked with dysgeusia.[4] Vismodegib, a first-in-class, small-molecule inhibitor of the hedgehog pathway produced dysgeusia in 51% of participants in a phase 1 trial for management of advanced basal cell carcinomas.[75]

OSTEONECROSIS OF THE JAWS

Bisphosphonates and denosumab (monoclonal antibody against receptor activator of nuclear factor kappa-B ligand) are antiresorptive medications that markedly slow bone turnover and remodeling and therefore increase bone density; they are used to treat postmenopausal osteoporosis and reduce skeletal-related events during cancer therapy (especially in patients with plasma cell myeloma and metastatic cancers).[76] Osteonecrosis is an ADE presenting as either exposed or nonexposed devitalized bone or a nonhealing extraction socket (**Fig. 8**).[77]

Antiangiogenic agents, such as bevacizumab and sunitinib, which act against vascular endothelial growth factor (VEGF), either used alone or in combination with bisphosphonates, also lead to the development of osteonecrosis in some patients.[78,79] The use of such anti-VEGF therapies

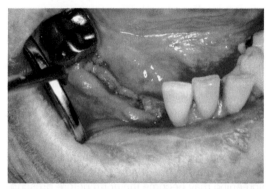

Fig. 8. Bisphosphonate-related osteonecrosis of the jaw: exposed bone of the right mandibular alveolar ridge.

and bisphosphonates in combination has demonstrated higher incidences of osteonecrosis (up to 10%) than with bisphosphonates alone.[80,81] The monoclonal antibody against VEGF receptor alibercept has been reported to cause osteonecrosis when used alone without bisphosphonates, radiation, or associated medications.[82] Other MTKIs, such as sorafenib, regorafenib, axinitinib, imatinib, nilotinib, and pazopanib, have also been implicated in nonantiresorptive medication-related osteonecrosis of the jaw.[83]

INFECTION

It is well-established that immunosuppressed patients frequently develop pseudomembranous candidiasis (**Fig. 9**), deep fungal infections, and viral infections.[84,85] TNF-α therapy specifically has been linked to osteomyelitis of the jaw,[86] and an increased risk of serious infections, such as tuberculosis and viral meningitis, especially when combined with other immunomodulatory agents.[87,88] Patients receiving infliximab and adalimumab were demonstrated to be at an increased

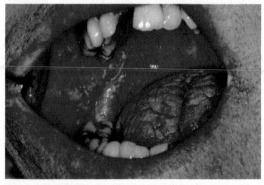

Fig. 9. Candidiasis from topical steroid therapy: white curdy papules and plaques on right buccal mucosa.

risk for tuberculosis (odds ratio, 2.0) and histoplasmosis and coccidiomycosis.[89] Disease-modifying antirheumatic drugs, such as methotrexate, abatacept, and alefacept, have been associated with herpes simplex or zoster, deep fungal infections, and tuberculosis.[90]

ANGIOEDEMA

Medication-induced angioedema has been observed with multiple agents, most commonly ACE inhibitors.[91] This abrupt onset swelling of the orofacial region and lips is mediated by inflammatory cytokines and complement activation, and results in vascular permeability; this may compromise the airway and be life-threatening. It has also been reported with the use of other antihypertensive agents, such as angiotensin receptor blockers, calcium channel blockers, and hydrochlorothiazide, and antiplatelet agents, such as thienopyridine and clopidogrel.[92,93] The use of the statin class of medications is infrequently associated with this side effect.[94]

MALIGNANCY AND LEUKOPLAKIA

Several chemotherapy and immunomodulating agents have been demonstrated to increase the risk of lymphoproliferative disorders and neoplasms.[95] Patients taking methotrexate for rheumatoid arthritis sometimes develop lymphoproliferative diseases that are often associated with Epstein-Barr virus, and approximately 20% regressed after discontinuation of the medication.[96,97]

Topical tacrolimus applied on the skin in a murine model exhibited development of cutaneous squamous cell carcinomas in 8.5% of cases and benign papillomas in 91.5% of cases.[98] There have been anecdotal reports of oral squamous cell carcinoma developing in patients with oral LP treated off-label with tacrolimus ointment.[99,100] Tacrolimus has been shown to have an effect on the MAPK and p53 pathways, which are important in cancer signaling.[100] In a long-term study of liver transplant recipients, 45% of de novo malignancies were on the skin, with tacrolimus immunosuppression cited as a risk factor (hazard ratio, 2.06).[101] There have been only sporadic case reports of squamous cell carcinomas of the skin and cutaneous T-cell lymphomas occurring after tacrolimus and pimecrolimus application.[102,103]

BRAF inhibitors, such as vemurafenib used to treat advanced melanoma, have been associated with the development of leukoplakia and cutaneous tumors lesions, such as verrucous keratoses[68] and squamous cell carcinomas.[104–106] It has also been reported that 9.6% of patients on combinations of immunomodulating agents, such as azathioprine, cyclophosphamide, cyclosporine, or mycophenolate mofetil for pemphigus or pemphigoid, may develop a secondary malignancy, such as skin, breast, or bladder cancer, and leukemia.[107]

Malignancies induced by biologic agents have been reported in the literature. Bongartz and colleagues[89] analyzed nine randomized, controlled trials of infliximab and adalimumab and found a three-fold increase of malignancy in patients treated with higher doses of anti-TNF antibodies, with most tumors comprised of basal cell carcinomas and lymphomas. However, another study evaluated 18 clinical trials using TNF-α inhibitors and found no increase in malignancy or infection.[108] The issue of drug-induced malignancy is still controversial and there may be confounding factors, such as immunodysregulation caused by the disease for which the drug is being given, leading to malignancy. Rheumatoid arthritis, for instance, is associated with the development of lymphoma regardless of therapy,[109] and the use of concomitant powerful immunosuppressive medications likely increases the risk.[110]

SUMMARY

ADEs in the oral cavity are common and may have a variety of clinical presentations. With new therapeutic agents being introduced into clinical practice, it is likely that more ADEs will be encountered. The advent of targeted therapies in oncology has produced several novel complications in the oral cavity. Health care providers should be aware of the manifestations of ADEs in their practice.

DISCLOSURE

The authors have nothing to disclose.

REFERENCES

1. Edwards IR, Aronson JK. Adverse drug reactions: definitions, diagnosis, and management. Lancet 2000;356(9237):1255–9.
2. Nebeker JR, Barach P, Samore MH. Clarifying adverse drug events: a clinician's guide to terminology, documentation, and reporting. Ann Intern Med 2004;140(10):795–801.
3. Wolff A, Joshi RK, Ekstrom J, et al. A guide to medications inducing salivary gland dysfunction, xerostomia, and subjective sialorrhea: a systematic review sponsored by the World Workshop on Oral Medicine VI. Drugs R D 2017;17(1):1–28.

4. Vigarios E, Epstein JB, Sibaud V. Oral mucosal changes induced by anticancer targeted therapies and immune checkpoint inhibitors. Support Care Cancer 2017;25(5):1713–39.
5. Ismail SB, Kumar SK, Zain RB. Oral lichen planus and lichenoid reactions: etiopathogenesis, diagnosis, management and malignant transformation. J Oral Sci 2007;49(2):89–106.
6. Breathnach SM. Mechanisms of drug eruptions: part I. Australas J Dermatol 1995;36(3):121–7.
7. Li D, Li J, Li C, et al. The association of thyroid disease and oral lichen planus: a literature review and meta-analysis. Front Endocrinol (Lausanne) 2017; 8:310.
8. Sugerman PB, Savage NW, Zhou X, et al. Oral lichen planus. Clin Dermatol 2000;18(5):533–9.
9. Schlosser BJ. Lichen planus and lichenoid reactions of the oral mucosa. Dermatol Ther 2010; 23(3):251–67.
10. Sibaud V, Eid C, Belum VR, et al. Oral lichenoid reactions associated with anti-PD-1/PD-L1 therapies: clinicopathological findings. J Eur Acad Dermatol Venereol 2017;31(10):e464–9.
11. Shazib MA, Woo SB, Sroussi H, et al. Oral immune-related adverse events associated with PD-1 inhibitor therapy: a case series. Oral Dis 2020;26(2): 325–33.
12. Pua VS, Scolyer RA, Barnetson RS. Pravastatin-induced lichenoid drug eruption. Australas J Dermatol 2006;47(1):57–9.
13. Vinay K, Yanamandra U, Dogra S, et al. Long-term mucocutaneous adverse effects of imatinib in Indian chronic myeloid leukemia patients. Int J Dermatol 2018;57(3):332–8.
14. Mann BS, Johnson JR, Kelly R, et al. Letrozole in the extended adjuvant treatment of postmenopausal women with history of early-stage breast cancer who have completed 5 years of adjuvant tamoxifen. Clin Cancer Res 2005; 11(16):5671–7.
15. Asarch A, Gottlieb AB, Lee J, et al. Lichen planus-like eruptions: an emerging side effect of tumor necrosis factor-alpha antagonists. J Am Acad Dermatol 2009;61(1):104–11.
16. Moss AC, Treister NS, Marsee DK, et al. Clinical challenges and images in GI. Oral lichenoid reaction in a patient with Crohn's disease receiving infliximab. Gastroenterology 2007;132(2):488, 829.
17. Mocciaro F, Orlando A, Renna S, et al. Oral lichen planus after certolizumab pegol treatment in a patient with Crohn's disease. J Crohns Colitis 2011; 5(2):173–4.
18. Fiorentino DF. The yin and yang of TNF-{alpha} inhibition. Arch Dermatol 2007;143(2):233–6.
19. Bakkour W, Coulson IH. GA101 (a novel anti-CD20 monoclonal antibody)-induced lichenoid eruption. Dermatol Ther (Heidelb) 2012;2(1):3.
20. Ozkaya E. Oral mucosal fixed drug eruption: characteristics and differential diagnosis. J Am Acad Dermatol 2013;69(2):e51–8.
21. Inamadar AC, Palit A, Athanikar SB, et al. Multiple fixed drug eruptions due to cetirizine. Br J Dermatol 2002;147(5):1025–6.
22. Mahajan VK, Sharma NL, Sharma VC. Fixed drug eruption: a novel side-effect of levocetirizine. Int J Dermatol 2005;44(9):796–8.
23. Mahendra A, Gupta S, Gupta S, et al. Oral fixed drug eruption due to fluconazole. Indian J Dermatol Venereol Leprol 2006;72(5):391.
24. Heikkila H, Timonen K, Stubb S. Fixed drug eruption due to fluconazole. J Am Acad Dermatol 2000;42(5 Pt 2):883–4.
25. Alonso JC, Melgosa AC, Gonzalo MJ, et al. Fixed drug eruption on the tongue due to clarithromycin. Contact Dermatitis 2005;53(2):121–2.
26. Gupta S, Gupta S, Mittal A, et al. Oral fixed drug eruption caused by gabapentin. J Eur Acad Dermatol Venereol 2009;23(10):1207–8.
27. Singh R, Ramachandra SS, Dayakara JK. Oral fixed drug eruption due to tinidazole. Cutis 2016; 98(6):E1–2.
28. Wong ITY, Huang Y, Zhou Y. Drug eruption to rosuvastatin with recurrence on simvastatin: a case report. J Cutan Med Surg 2018;22(3):359–61.
29. Klimi E. A probable case of mucosal fixed drug eruption following treatment with silodosin. Sultan Qaboos Univ Med J 2018;18(3):e402–4.
30. Boulinguez S, Reix S, Bedane C, et al. Role of drug exposure in aphthous ulcers: a case-control study. Br J Dermatol 2000;143(6):1261–5.
31. Bagan JV, Thongprasom K, Scully C. Adverse oral reactions associated with the COX-2 inhibitor rofecoxib. Oral Dis 2004;10(6):401–3.
32. Goffin E, Pochet JM, Lejuste P, et al. Aphtous ulcers of the mouth associated with losartan. Clin Nephrol 1998;50(3):197.
33. Martins F, de Oliveira MA, Wang Q, et al. A review of oral toxicity associated with mTOR inhibitor therapy in cancer patients. Oral Oncol 2013;49(4): 293–8.
34. de Oliveira MA, Martins EMF, Wang Q, et al. Clinical presentation and management of mTOR inhibitor-associated stomatitis. Oral Oncol 2011; 47(10):998–1003.
35. Sonis ST. Regimen-related gastrointestinal toxicities in cancer patients. Curr Opin Support Palliat Care 2010;4(1):26–30.
36. Philipone E, Rockafellow A, Sternberg R, et al. Oral ulcerations as a sequela of tacrolimus and mycophenolate mofetil therapy. Oral Surg Oral Med Oral Pathol Oral Radiol 2014;118(6):e175–8.
37. Mignogna MD, Fortuna G, Leuci S, et al. Sunitinib adverse event: oral bullous and lichenoid mucositis. Ann Pharmacother 2009;43(3):546–7.

38. Baum S, Sakka N, Artsi O, et al. Diagnosis and classification of autoimmune blistering diseases. Autoimmun Rev 2014;13(4–5):482–9.

39. Weller R, White MI. Bullous pemphigoid and penicillamine. Clin Exp Dermatol 1996;21(2):121–2.

40. Matz H, Bialy-Golan A, Brenner S. Diclofenac: a new trigger of pemphigus vulgaris? Dermatology 1997;195(1):48–9.

41. Vassileva S. Drug-induced pemphigoid: bullous and cicatricial. Clin Dermatol 1998;16(3):379–87.

42. Stavropoulos PG, Soura E, Antoniou C. Drug-induced pemphigoid: a review of the literature. J Eur Acad Dermatol Venereol 2014;28(9):1133–40.

43. Naidoo J, Schindler K, Querfeld C, et al. Autoimmune bullous skin disorders with immune checkpoint inhibitors targeting PD-1 and PD-L1. Cancer Immunol Res 2016;4(5):383–9.

44. Edwards D, Boritz E, Cowen EW, et al. Erythema multiforme major following treatment with infliximab. Oral Surg Oral Med Oral Pathol Oral Radiol 2013;115(2):e36–40.

45. Salama M, Lawrance IC. Stevens-Johnson syndrome complicating adalimumab therapy in Crohn's disease. World J Gastroenterol 2009;15(35):4449–52.

46. Taqi SA. Drug-induced oral erythema multiforme: a diagnostic challenge. Ann Afr Med 2018;17(1):43–5.

47. Auquier-Dunant A, Mockenhaupt M, Naldi L, et al. Correlations between clinical patterns and causes of erythema multiforme majus, Stevens-Johnson syndrome, and toxic epidermal necrolysis: results of an international prospective study. Arch Dermatol 2002;138(8):1019–24.

48. Goldinger SM, Stieger P, Meier B, et al. Cytotoxic cutaneous adverse drug reactions during anti-PD-1 therapy. Clin Cancer Res 2016;22(16):4023–9.

49. Miliszewski MA, Kirchhof MG, Sikora S, et al. Stevens-Johnson syndrome and toxic epidermal necrolysis: an analysis of triggers and implications for improving prevention. Am J Med 2016;129(11):1221–5.

50. Hung SI, Chung WH, Jee SH, et al. Genetic susceptibility to carbamazepine-induced cutaneous adverse drug reactions. Pharmacogenet Genomics 2006;16(4):297–306.

51. Yu KH, Yu CY, Fang YF. Diagnostic utility of HLA-B*5801 screening in severe allopurinol hypersensitivity syndrome: an updated systematic review and meta-analysis. Int J Rheum Dis 2017;20(9):1057–71.

52. Gerogianni K, Tsezou A, Dimas K. Drug-induced skin adverse reactions: the role of pharmacogenomics in their prevention. Mol Diagn Ther 2018;22(3):297–314.

53. Lerman MA, Karimbux N, Guze KA, et al. Pigmentation of the hard palate. Oral Surg Oral Med Oral Pathol Oral Radiol Endod 2009;107(1):8–12.

54. Tosios KI, Kalogirou EM, Sklavounou A. Drug-associated hyperpigmentation of the oral mucosa: report of four cases. Oral Surg Oral Med Oral Pathol Oral Radiol 2018;125(3):e54–66.

55. Arora B, Kumar L, Sharma A, et al. Pigmentary changes in chronic myeloid leukemia patients treated with imatinib mesylate. Ann Oncol 2004;15(2):358–9.

56. Scully C, Bagan JV. Adverse drug reactions in the orofacial region. Crit Rev Oral Biol Med 2004;15(4):221–39.

57. Stahli BE, Schwab S. Amiodarone-induced skin hyperpigmentation. QJM 2011;104(8):723–4.

58. Molina-Ruiz AM, Pulpillo A, Molina-Ruiz RM, et al. Chlorpromazine-induced severe skin pigmentation and corneal opacities in a patient with schizophrenia. Int J Dermatol 2016;55(8):909–12.

59. Seymour RA, Thomason JM, Ellis JS. The pathogenesis of drug-induced gingival overgrowth. J Clin Periodontol 1996;23(3 Pt 1):165–75.

60. Brown RS, Arany PR. Mechanism of drug-induced gingival overgrowth revisited: a unifying hypothesis. Oral Dis 2015;21(1):e51–61.

61. Woo SB, Allen CM, Orden A, et al. Non-gingival soft tissue growths after allogeneic marrow transplantation. Bone Marrow Transplant 1996;17(6):1127–32.

62. Al-Mohaya M, Treister N, Al-Khadra O, et al. Calcineurin inhibitor-associated oral inflammatory polyps after transplantation. J Oral Pathol Med 2007;36(9):570–4.

63. Bostanci N, Ilgenli T, Pirhan DC, et al. Relationship between IL-1A polymorphisms and gingival overgrowth in renal transplant recipients receiving cyclosporin A. J Clin Periodontol 2006;33(11):771–8.

64. Le QT, Kim HE, Schneider CJ, et al. Palifermin reduces severe mucositis in definitive chemoradiotherapy of locally advanced head and neck cancer: a randomized, placebo-controlled study. J Clin Oncol 2011;29(20):2808–14.

65. Lauritano D, Petruzzi M, Di Stasio D, et al. Clinical effectiveness of palifermin in prevention and treatment of oral mucositis in children with acute lymphoblastic leukaemia: a case-control study. Int J Oral Sci 2014;6(1):27–30.

66. Lerman MA, Treister NS. Generalized white appearance of the oral mucosa. Hyperkeratosis secondary to palifermin. J Am Dent Assoc 2010;141(7):867–9.

67. Spielberger R, Stiff P, Bensinger W, et al. Palifermin for oral mucositis after intensive therapy for hematologic cancers. N Engl J Med 2004;351(25):2590–8.

68. Ganzenmueller T, Hage E, Yakushko Y, et al. No human virus sequences detected by next-generation

sequencing in benign verrucous skin tumors occurring in BRAF-inhibitor-treated patients. Exp Dermatol 2013;22(11):725–9.

69. Dorchin M, Masoumi Dehshiri R, Soleiman S, et al. Evaluation of neuropathy during intensive vincristine chemotherapy for non-Hodgkin's lymphoma and acute lymphoblastic leukemia. Iran J Ped Hematol Oncol 2013;3(4):138–42.

70. Tuccori M, Lapi F, Testi A, et al. Drug-induced taste and smell alterations: a case/non-case evaluation of an Italian database of spontaneous adverse drug reaction reporting. Drug Saf 2011;34(10):849–59.

71. Han Y, Smith MT. Pathobiology of cancer chemotherapy-induced peripheral neuropathy (CIPN). Front Pharmacol 2013;4:156.

72. Park SB, Goldstein D, Krishnan AV, et al. Chemotherapy-induced peripheral neurotoxicity: a critical analysis. CA Cancer J Clin 2013;63(6):419–37.

73. Yuan A, Kurtz SL, Barysauskas CM, et al. Oral adverse events in cancer patients treated with VEGFR-directed multitargeted tyrosine kinase inhibitors. Oral Oncol 2015;51(11):1026–33.

74. Kollmannsberger C, Bjarnason G, Burnett P, et al. Sunitinib in metastatic renal cell carcinoma: recommendations for management of noncardiovascular toxicities. Oncologist 2011;16(5):543–53.

75. Sekulic A, Migden MR, Oro AE, et al. Efficacy and safety of vismodegib in advanced basal-cell carcinoma. N Engl J Med 2012;366(23):2171–9.

76. Woo SB, Hellstein JW, Kalmar JR. Narrative [corrected] review: bisphosphonates and osteonecrosis of the jaws. Ann Intern Med 2006;144(10):753–61.

77. Ruggiero SL, Dodson TB, Fantasia J, et al. American Association of Oral and Maxillofacial Surgeons position paper on medication-related osteonecrosis of the jaw: 2014 update. J Oral Maxillofac Surg 2014;72(10):1938–56.

78. Nicolatou-Galitis O, Migkou M, Psyrri A, et al. Gingival bleeding and jaw bone necrosis in patients with metastatic renal cell carcinoma receiving sunitinib: report of 2 cases with clinical implications. Oral Surg Oral Med Oral Pathol Oral Radiol 2012;113(2):234–8.

79. Estilo CL, Fornier M, Farooki A, et al. Osteonecrosis of the jaw related to bevacizumab. J Clin Oncol 2008;26(24):4037–8.

80. Smidt-Hansen T, Folkmar TB, Fode K, et al. Combination of zoledronic acid and targeted therapy is active but may induce osteonecrosis of the jaw in patients with metastatic renal cell carcinoma. J Oral Maxillofac Surg 2013;71(9):1532–40.

81. Christodoulou C, Pervena A, Klouvas G, et al. Combination of bisphosphonates and antiangiogenic factors induces osteonecrosis of the jaw more frequently than bisphosphonates alone. Oncology 2009;76(3):209–11.

82. Zarringhalam P, Brizman E, Shakib K. Medication-related osteonecrosis of the jaw associated with aflibercept. Br J Oral Maxillofac Surg 2017;55(3):314–5.

83. Nicolatou-Galitis O, Kouri M, Papadopoulou E, et al. Osteonecrosis of the jaw related to non-antiresorptive medications: a systematic review. Support Care Cancer 2019;27(2):383–94.

84. Marsot-Dupuch K, Quillard J, Meyohas MC. Head and neck lesions in the immunocompromised host. Eur Radiol 2004;14(Suppl 3):E155–67.

85. Samonis G, Mantadakis E, Maraki S. Orofacial viral infections in the immunocompromised host. Oncol Rep 2000;7(6):1389–94.

86. Teshima CW, Thompson A, Dhanoa L, et al. Long-term response rates to infliximab therapy for Crohn's disease in an outpatient cohort. Can J Gastroenterol 2009;23(5):348–52.

87. Deepak P, Stobaugh DJ, Ehrenpreis ED. Infectious complications of TNF-alpha inhibitor monotherapy versus combination therapy with immunomodulators in inflammatory bowel disease: analysis of the Food and Drug Administration Adverse Event Reporting System. J Gastrointestin Liver Dis 2013;22(3):269–76.

88. Delabaye I, De Keyser F. 74-week follow-up of safety of infliximab in patients with refractory rheumatoid arthritis. Arthritis Res Ther 2010;12(3):R121.

89. Bongartz T, Sutton AJ, Sweeting MJ, et al. Anti-TNF antibody therapy in rheumatoid arthritis and the risk of serious infections and malignancies: systematic review and meta-analysis of rare harmful effects in randomized controlled trials. JAMA 2006;295(19):2275–85.

90. Salvana EM, Salata RA. Infectious complications associated with monoclonal antibodies and related small molecules. Clin Microbiol Rev 2009;22(2):274–90.

91. Hom KA, Hirsch R, Elluru RG. Antihypertensive drug-induced angioedema causing upper airway obstruction in children. Int J Pediatr Otorhinolaryngol 2012;76(1):14–9.

92. Shino M, Takahashi K, Murata T, et al. Angiotensin II receptor blocker-induced angioedema in the oral floor and epiglottis. Am J Otolaryngol 2011;32(6):624–6.

93. Ruscin JM, Page RL 2nd, Scott J. Hydrochlorothiazide-induced angioedema in a patient allergic to sulfonamide antibiotics: evidence from a case report and a review of the literature. Am J Geriatr Pharmacother 2006;4(4):325–9.

94. Nisly SAAK, Knight TB. Simvastatin: a risk factor for angioedema? J Pharm Technol 2013;29:149–52.

95. Bagg A, Dunphy CH. Immunosuppressive and immunomodulatory   therapy-associated

lymphoproliferative disorders. Semin Diagn Pathol 2013;30(2):102–12.

96. Hoshida Y, Xu JX, Fujita S, et al. Lymphoproliferative disorders in rheumatoid arthritis: clinicopathological analysis of 76 cases in relation to methotrexate medication. J Rheumatol 2007; 34(2):322–31.

97. Ichikawa A, Arakawa F, Kiyasu J, et al. Methotrexate/iatrogenic lymphoproliferative disorders in rheumatoid arthritis: histology, Epstein-Barr virus, and clonality are important predictors of disease progression and regression. Eur J Haematol 2013;91(1):20–8.

98. Niwa Y, Terashima T, Sumi H. Topical application of the immunosuppressant tacrolimus accelerates carcinogenesis in mouse skin. Br J Dermatol 2003;149(5):960–7.

99. Mattsson U, Magnusson B, Jontell M. Squamous cell carcinoma in a patient with oral lichen planus treated with topical application of tacrolimus. Oral Surg Oral Med Oral Pathol Oral Radiol Endod 2010;110(1):e19–25.

100. Becker JC, Houben R, Vetter CS, et al. The carcinogenic potential of tacrolimus ointment beyond immune suppression: a hypothesis creating case report. BMC Cancer 2006;6:7.

101. Wimmer CD, Angele MK, Schwarz B, et al. Impact of cyclosporine versus tacrolimus on the incidence of de novo malignancy following liver transplantation: a single center experience with 609 patients. Transpl Int 2013;26(10):999–1006.

102. Berger TG, Duvic M, Van Voorhees AS, et al. The use of topical calcineurin inhibitors in dermatology: safety concerns. Report of the American Academy of Dermatology Association Task Force. J Am Acad Dermatol 2006;54(5):818–23.

103. Tennis P, Gelfand JM, Rothman KJ. Evaluation of cancer risk related to atopic dermatitis and use of topical calcineurin inhibitors. Br J Dermatol 2011; 165(3):465–73.

104. Vigarios E, Lamant L, Delord JP, et al. Oral squamous cell carcinoma and hyperkeratotic lesions with BRAF inhibitors. Br J Dermatol 2015;172(6): 1680–2.

105. Pileri A, Cricca M, Gandolfi L, et al. Vemurafenib mucosal side-effect. J Eur Acad Dermatol Venereol 2016;30(6):1053–5.

106. Holderfield M, Deuker MM, McCormick F, et al. Targeting RAF kinases for cancer therapy: BRAF-mutated melanoma and beyond. Nat Rev Cancer 2014;14(7):455–67.

107. Mabrouk D, Gurcan HM, Keskin DB, et al. Association between cancer and immunosuppressive therapy: analysis of selected studies in pemphigus and pemphigoid. Ann Pharmacother 2010;44(11): 1770–6.

108. Leombruno JP, Einarson TR, Keystone EC. The safety of anti-tumour necrosis factor treatments in rheumatoid arthritis: meta and exposure-adjusted pooled analyses of serious adverse events. Ann Rheum Dis 2009;68(7):1136–45.

109. Baecklund E, Backlin C, Iliadou A, et al. Characteristics of diffuse large B cell lymphomas in rheumatoid arthritis. Arthritis Rheum 2006;54(12):3774–81.

110. Mawardi H, Elad S, Correa ME, et al. Oral epithelial dysplasia and squamous cell carcinoma following allogeneic hematopoietic stem cell transplantation: clinical presentation and treatment outcomes. Bone Marrow Transplant 2011;46(6):884–91.

Dental Considerations in Patients with Oral Mucosal Diseases

Wesley Sherrell, DMD[a],*, Bhavik Desai, DMD, PhD[b],
Thomas P. Sollecito, DMD, FDS RCSEd[c]

KEYWORDS

- Dental considerations • Oral mucosal diseases • Topical agents • Malignant transformation
- Caries risk and prevention

KEY POINTS

- To improve outcomes in patients with mucocutaneous disease.
- To inform the dermatologist of oral mucosal disease implication on dental health and overall oral health.
- To help the dermatologist guide both the patient and the oral health care provider in the appropriate dental care regimen among this complex patient population.

INTRODUCTION

Oral mucosal diseases are a significant health care burden in medical and dental practices.[1] Other articles of this issue include specific oral mucosal diseases commonly encountered in dermatologic practices. This article focuses on the dental health in patients with conditions such as oral lichen planus, mucous membrane pemphigoid, and oral mucosal disorders related to systemic diseases. An appreciation of the dental condition by dermatologists and the mucocutaneous condition by the dentist will lead to improved dental and mucocutaneous outcomes. The aim of this article is to inform dermatologists of the implications that oral mucosal diseases exert on the dental condition to help the dermatologist guide both the patient and the dental provider in appropriate management of this complex patient population.

CHALLENGES WITH HOME CARE IN THE PATIENT WITH MUCOCUTANEOUS DISEASE

Patients with oral mucosal disease face several challenges with dental care and maintenance of

adequate oral hygiene.[2] Inflammatory oral lesions, including oral lichen planus, oral hypersensitivity reactions and other mucocutaneous disorders, often present with pain which may impede the patient's ability to maintain adequate oral hygiene. Oral pain, including burning from mucosal diseases, has been associated with a diminished quality of life.[3] Oral vesiculobullous lesions can lead to ulceration and bleeding, further aggravating painful oral symptoms.[4] Discomfort owing to thinning and bleeding of periodontal tissues can result in patients decreasing maintenance of their oral hygiene. Inadequate home care and maintenance of gingival and dental hygiene can result in the accumulation of local irritants, plaque, and calculus, leading to additional inflammation of the periodontal tissues affected by oral mucosal diseases.[5]

Hence, the presence of oral mucosal disease and the associated inability of patients to maintain adequate oral hygiene may worsen the prognosis of their dental and gingival health. Dental hygiene and prophylaxis may be required at more frequent intervals than the conventional protocol of every

[a] Oral Medicine, Division of Diagnostic Sciences, University of North Carolina Adams School of Dentistry, Campus Box #7450, Chapel Hill, NC 27599-7450, USA; [b] Private Practice, Affiliated Health of Wisconsin, Milwaukee, WI, USA; [c] Department of Oral Medicine, University of Pennsylvania School of Dental Medicine, 240 South 40th Street, Suite 200, Philadelphia, PA 19104, USA
* Corresponding author.
E-mail address: wesley_sherrell@unc.edu

Dermatol Clin 38 (2020) 535–541
https://doi.org/10.1016/j.det.2020.05.013

6 months, in individuals deemed to have a higher risk for periodontal disease.[6] For these reasons, patients with oral mucosal disease may require dental prophylaxis at increased frequency.

CHALLENGES WITH DENTAL TREATMENT IN THE PATIENT WITH MUCOCUTANEOUS DISEASE

Delivering dental care to patients with oral mucosal disease can present several challenges to dental professionals. A general understanding of dental treatment and its impact on mucosal disease by the dermatologist can help the dermatologist inform the dentist of important modifications, which should be considered in the provision of dental care.

Treatment Planning

Patients suffering from chronic mucosal diseases often receive modified dental treatment plans to accommodate their unique oral condition and dental needs. Patients with oral mucosal diseases are often managed with systemic medications, which may include corticosteroids, hydroxychloroquine, mycophenolate mofetil, azathioprine, mercaptopurine, monoclonal antibodies, and/or intravenous immunoglobulins. In patients using these medications, dentists may need to consider additional precautions to plan dental treatment. The sequencing of invasive dental procedures like extractions, gingival and periodontal surgeries, oral and maxillofacial surgeries, and dental implant placement may be altered if patients are on systemic immunosuppressive therapy to maximize potential for normal wound healing.[7] Hence, dental professionals are encouraged to consult with the patient's dermatologist and obtain the overall dermatologic treatment plan. Long-term topical steroid therapy, often prescribed for many oral mucosal diseases, may result in the potential thinning of the oral epithelium,[8] warranting an alternative dental treatment plan.

During Dental Treatment

Dental treatment may need to be delayed until symptoms and alterations caused by the oral mucosal disease are adequately controlled. For example, gingival enlargement or friability may interfere with dental procedures[9] by obstruction of the visual field and hindering placement of dental armamentarium such as rubber dams and/or matrix bands. Thinning of oral mucosa observed in vesiculobullous diseases may result in excessive bleeding and desquamation of epithelial tissue in the operative field, posing procedural challenges to dentists trying to achieve isolation from moisture, which is essential for optimum restorative dentistry.[10] Dental procedures are associated with a risk of iatrogenic injuries,[11] compounded by the active mucosal disease. Erosive lesions on the buccal mucosa and gingival tissue may result in increased patient discomfort during the dental procedures and may have to be delayed until asymptomatic and tissue healing has occurred. Severely symptomatic lesions may also restrict the dentist's ability to manipulate oral tissues for dental procedures. Desquamated oral epithelial tissue may become severely traumatized by high-speed dental suction, dental air/water syringes, and dental handpieces.

Caution also needs to be exerted during placement of sutures and application of caustic hemostatic agents such as silver nitrate to control bleeding in areas of active oral mucosal lesions.

After Dental Treatment

There is limited evidence suggesting oral mucosal disease has no major impact on wound healing secondary to periodontal surgery,[12] but caution should be exercised when planning invasive procedures on the oral tissues affected by mucosal disease. Topical preparations may require temporary discontinuance during the postprocedural healing phase.

THE DENTIST'S ROLE IN INTERDISCIPLINARY CARE OF THE PATIENT WITH MUCOCUTANEOUS DISEASE

Based on their extensive understanding of the anatomy and physiology of oral cavity, dental professionals play a key role in the interdisciplinary care of patients with oral mucosal diseases.

Management of Oral Signs and Symptoms with Topical Immunosuppressive Therapy

Topical steroids and other topical immunosuppressive agents, such as tacrolimus and azathioprine, have shown varying degrees of usefulness in the management of oral mucosal lesions.[13] Topical management of these conditions has been addressed in detail in other articles in this issue. Dental professionals may fabricate special medication trays for gingival tissues affected by the mucocutaneous disease. Such medication trays have been shown to successfully manage inflammation by placing the topical agent to the affected areas and placing the tray over the teeth covering the affected mucosa, acting as an occlusive dressing.[14]

Dental Evaluation Before Immunosuppressive Therapy

Before the start of systemic immunosuppressive therapy, medical providers rely on dentists to eliminate foci of oral odontogenic infection secondary to dental caries, dental periapical/pericoronal infections, and periodontal disease. The elimination of odontogenic infection has been associated with better prognosis of systemic therapy and more favorable health outcomes in other immunocompromised states, such as organ transplantation,[15] stem cell transplantation, and chemotherapy.[16]

Evidence-based clinical practice guidelines for dental clearance before the initiation of immunosuppressive drugs for mucocutaneous diseases are not available. However, it is not only important to treat infection in any circumstance, it may be postulated that elimination of oral foci of potential infections may result in better outcomes in patients before the initiation of systemic immunosuppressive therapy for mucocutaneous disease.

Professional Dental Prophylaxis and Oral Cancer Surveillance

As noted elsewhere in this article, adequate maintenance of oral hygiene may become challenging in patients with severely symptomatic oral mucosal diseases. Dermatologists may consider recommending more frequent dental hygiene visits for patients with oral mucosal diseases. Monitoring patients with oral mucosal diseases by the dentist also provides an opportunity to periodically evaluate the status of their mucosal disease and monitor the oral cavity for any precancerous and cancerous changes, such as epithelial dysplasia, carcinoma in situ, and oral squamous cell carcinoma or the development of lymphoma.

ORAL CONSIDERATIONS OF MEDICATIONS USED FOR THE MANAGEMENT OF MUCOCUTANEOUS DISEASES

With any medical therapy, there is a potential for adverse effects and complications. Both topical and systemic preparations used in the management of mucocutaneous diseases could have both acute and chronic effects, which may be localized or systemic in nature.

Local Penetration of Topical Agents

Penetration of topical agents used to manage oral mucosal diseases can be challenging owing to the presence of saliva in its ability to dilute or "wash-away" topical medications. Equally challenging in using topical preparations orally is that much of the oral mucosa is moveable and in contact with other structures in the mouth, which displaces the topical agent. For instance, the lateral tongue constantly contacts the mandibular teeth, which may dissolve any topical agents applied to that site. To enhance penetration, the medium of the topical agent used and the instructions given to the patient on how to properly apply it are critically important.[17] The preferred vehicle for the oral cavity is that of a gel for localized lesions and rinses for generalized lesions. Gels adhere to the mucosa more effectively than creams or ointments and they also have greater absorption into the oral mucosa owing to increased solubility.[18] Patients should be instructed to apply the agent to the affected site and then cover the area with gauze to prevent it being washed or wiped away. Rinses should be swished around the oral cavity for about 1 to 2 minutes, ensuring all affected sites are exposed and then the rinse should be expectorated to minimize systemic absorption. There are certain indications in which the rinse may be swallowed, such as in patients where systemic absorption is desired or in those who may have oropharyngeal or esophageal lesions.

Although systemic absorption of topical agents is significantly less compared with oral agents, it still should be taken into consideration and discussed with the patient when prescribing these therapies because they have the potential to induce hypothalamic–pituitary axis suppression. Systemic absorption of topical agents (henceforth systemic side effects) becomes more of a concern in patients who are using these agents on a chronic, frequent basis or inappropriately using too much medication. Furthermore, the greater the potency of the topical steroid, the greater the risk of systemic absorption and side effects.[17] For example, clobetasol would have a much higher potential for systemic absorption than triamcinolone.

Application of topical steroids in highly permeable areas, such as the mouth and in areas where the skin/mucosal barrier is damaged (as is frequently the case in oral mucosal disease), predisposes the patient to absorption and the systemic effects of steroids such as hypothalamic–pituitary axis suppression and hyperglycemia.[17,19] Children are at increased risk for hypothalamic–pituitary axis suppression and other systemic effects of ultrahigh-potency topical steroids given that their skin/mucosa is generally thinner and more permeable than that of adults.[17,19]

Adverse Drug Reactions

Medications, either topical or systemic, used to treat oral mucosal diseases have the potential to initiate allergic responses and hypersensitivity reactions. The sensitizing agent in the topical preparation is often not the active medication itself, but rather the transport vehicle or a preservative agent used in the preparation.[20,21] Patch testing can be used to determine whether the reaction is from the therapeutic agent, vehicle, or preservative.[21]

Acute adverse reactions of systemic steroids can include nausea, vomiting, rash, hives, itching, restlessness, hyperglycemia, and swelling of the face, lips, and tongue.[22] Other glucocorticoid-sparing systemic immunosuppressive agents commonly used to treat oral mucosal disease, such as mycophenolate mofetil, may have many of the same acute effects as systemic steroids, including allergic reactions, but their most common adverse effect is persistent diarrhea.[23]

Nonsteroidal anti-inflammatory drugs have also been implicated by multiple studies to cause lichenoid tissue reactions and therefore a patient with a diagnosis of a lichenoid tissue reaction who regularly uses nonsteroidal anti-inflammatory drugs, should eliminate the agent for a trial period and then been evaluated for improvement of the lichenoid reaction.[24]

All immunosuppressive agents used to treat oral mucosal diseases have the potential to make a patient susceptible to acute infections, both locally in the oral cavity and systemically, when using a systemic agent.

Dapsone, an antibacterial drug used to treat leprosy, has anti-inflammatory properties, and therefore is occasionally used to treat mucocutaneous diseases that are resistant to topical therapies and other systemic immunosuppressive therapies.[25,26] It has been shown to be efficacious in the management of both mucous membrane pemphigoid as well as pemphigus vulgaris.[25] Dapsone has the potential for serious adverse reactions, most notably being the development of hemolytic anemia in patients with glucose-6-phosphate-dehydrogenase (G6PD) deficiency.[26] For this reason, a G6PD deficiency screen should be completed before initiating any patient on dapsone.

Doxycycline and other tetracycline-based medications have multiple implications for mucocutaneous diseases affecting the oral cavity owing to their anti-inflammatory properties.[27] For this reason, they are commonly used as a treatment modality for certain mucosal diseases, such as mucous membrane pemphigoid.[27] Doxycycline is also an effective agent used in the management of periodontal disease. It is commonly used at subantimicrobial doses for this purpose.[27] One adverse effect of the tetracyclines that is common is staining of teeth and underlying alveolar bone. This effect is more common and pronounced in children because their teeth are developing, but it may occur in adults as well.[28]

Drug–Drug Interactions

There are potential drug–drug interactions among medications commonly used for dental diseases and medications used to manage mucocutaneous disease. Oral health care providers commonly prescribe antibiotics to treat infection, nonsteroidal anti-inflammatory drugs and narcotics to manage acute pain, and antimicrobial rinses such as chlorhexidine gluconate to manage periodontal disease. Several antibiotics that may be prescribed by oral health care providers such as clarithromycin, erythromycin, metronidazole, trimethoprim/sulfamethoxazole (Bactrim), and ciprofloxacin all inhibit the hepatic cytochrome p450 enzymes.[29] Therefore, the potential for adverse reactions exist if other medications which are metabolized by cytochrome p450 such as fluconazole,[30] which is occasionally prescribed for prophylaxis against candida in patients using immunosuppressive agents. Fluconazole for candida infections should also be used with caution in patients taking warfarin and β-hydroxy β-methylglutaryl coenzyme A reductase inhibitor medications as fluconazole may lead to dangerously elevated blood levels of these medications.[30]

Nonsteroidal anti-inflammatory drugs are commonly used to manage pain by oral health care professionals. One common side effect of these drugs is gastrointestinal upset, which is also a common side effect of common immunosuppressive medications used to manage mucocutaneous disease, such as prednisone and mycophenolate mofetil.[23]

Monitoring for Malignant Transformation

There are several immunomodulating medications that have been either reported to or shown to increase the risk of lymphoma.[31] Topical tacrolimus is a calcineurin inhibitor that is commonly used off-label in the management of mucocutaneous diseases. There have been a few case reports that have reported topical tacrolimus being associated with cutaneous T-cell lymphoma formation, but this association has never been definitively proven.[32–34] Given its efficacy in treating oral mucosal diseases that are resistant to topical steroid therapy, the clinician should be aware of the rare cases of it potentially being associated with malignancy.[32] There are reports in the literature, including a meta-analysis completed by Bongartz and colleagues,[35] of malignancies caused by biologic agents which showed a 3-fold increase in malignancy in patients using adalimumab and infliximab.[32] The malignancies cited in this study were mostly basal cell carcinomas and lymphomas.[32,35] It is worth noting that there are mucocutaneous diseases associated with autoimmune conditions, which increase the risk of a patient developing malignancies. Rheumatoid arthritis, Sjogren's syndrome, and systemic lupus have been associated with the development of lymphoma, including the potential for lymphoma within the oral cavity.[36]

There are multiple chemotherapeutic and immunomodulating therapies that have been reported to increase the chance of developing a malignancy. In a study using a murine model, topical tacrolimus was applied to the skin it was also shown that the subjects developed squamous cell carcinomas in 8.5% of cases and benign papillomas in 91.5% of cases.[32,37] This progression has never been exhibited in a human model. Furthermore, in the murine model, the mice were shaved, and large portions of their bodies were covered in the tacrolimus.[37] Several immunomodulating therapies when used in combination in the management of pemphigus and pemphigoid have been reported to cause a nonmelanoma skin cancer. These therapies include combinations of mycophenolate mofetil, cyclosporine, cyclophosphamide, or azathioprine.[32,38]

Certain oral mucosal diseases, such as lichen planus and lichenoid mucositis, have the potential to undergo malignant transformation. The risk for malignant transformation varies based on the study cited, but the most widely accepted value is about a 1% malignant transformation rate for lichen planus.[39] The overwhelming majority of these cases are on the lateral border of the tongue and occur in the erosive form of the disease. Therefore, monitoring the oral cavity in patients with an oral lichenoid reaction is important because early detection results in better outcomes.[40]

Oral Infections

Systemic agents such as prednisone, mycophenolate, and biologic agents will suppress the patient's overall ability to mount an immune response, thereby increasing a patient's risk of developing a variety of infections. Chronically immunosuppressed patients may require the use of prophylactic use of agents such as an antifungal agent.[39]

Topical steroids effectively decrease local immunity by means of vasoconstriction thereby preventing inflammatory immunogenic cells from reaching the tissues. The amount of vasoconstriction and henceforth the expected decrease in local immunity depends on the potency of the topical steroid used. Ultrahigh potency steroids such as clobetasol exert the greatest amount of vasoconstriction and therefore the most significant amount of immune suppression.[17] This decrease in local immunity often allows for opportunistic organisms such as *Candida* species to overgrow leading to candida infection. Candidiasis of the oral cavity and oropharynx is a very common condition; approximately 60% of the population have *Candida* living commensally without clinical manifestations.[41,42] When the immune system's ability to function becomes altered, such as in the use of topical steroids or with use of systemic immunosuppressive agents, fungal organisms have the opportunity to overgrow and have clinical consequences. For these reasons, many clinicians use topical antifungal agents such as nystatin oral suspension or clotrimazole troches in a prophylactic fashion for patients who are on chronic topical and systemic immunosuppressive therapies.[39]

Caries Risk and Prevention

A common side effect of many systemic medications is the disturbance of salivary function, leading to salivary hypofunction. Saliva fulfills many vital roles within the oral cavity, one of which is protecting the teeth from demineralization leading to cavitation of the tooth structure, otherwise known as dental decay or dental caries.[43] Saliva provides protection of caries by acting as a natural buffering solution for the acid produced by the cariogenic bacteria in the oral cavity as well as the acid ingested as a part of the human diet.[43] Saliva also physically washes away carbohydrates from teeth, denying the cariogenic bacteria of a substrate needed to produce acid that causes tooth demineralization and caries.[43] Therefore, by decreasing the saliva produced, certain medications can greatly increase the risk of dental caries.

Furthermore, topical medications used to treat oral mucosal disease or prevent oral candidiasis, such as nystatin, contain highly fermentable sugars. This ingredient can greatly increase a patient's caries risk, because patients use these agents multiple times per day while being instructed to have nothing by mouth for 30 minutes after applying the agent. The dentition is exposed to fermentable sugars for long periods of time. To mitigate the increased caries risk, topical agents can be made without fermentable sugar. These specialized preparations are not readily available at many retail pharmacies and in many instances have to be filled at a compounding pharmacy who can eliminate the fermentable sugar component.

Another important consideration in the prevention of caries in this population is use of fluoride. Fluoride has been proven to have a protective effect against dental caries. It is essential that patients who are at a high risk of caries, such as those who have xerostomia, and using topical preparations with fermentable sugar have adequate fluoride exposure. For this reason, many of these patients are given a prescription toothpaste with higher concentrations of fluoride.

SUMMARY

The population of complex patients who present with oral mucosal manifestations of mucocutaneous diseases require a team of practitioners working in conjunction to properly manage these patients. The dermatologist, the oral medicine specialist, the dentist, and the dental hygienist are all integral components of this team. It is essential for the dermatologist to be aware of a patient's dental health and overall oral condition. It is crucial to consider the unique environment of the oral cavity including the presence of saliva and exposure of food products when selecting appropriate therapies. The dermatologist needs to be mindful of oral infection exacerbation by the inability to maintain proper oral hygiene or by the use of immunosuppressive agents to treat the mucocutaneous disease. The dermatologist should also recognize the potential for these agents (or the underlying mucocutaneous disease itself) to be associated with malignant transformation. When using systemic therapies, it is paramount to consider their dental implications as well as their potential for interaction among other medications often prescribed for the dental patient. The dermatologist should expect the dental team to aid in the fabrication of medication trays to enhance topical medication delivery. Last, it is important to recognize that the highly fermentable sugars that are in some topical preparations used to treat oral mucosal disease are associated with a greater caries risk and coordination with the dental team for more frequent dental examination and topical fluoride supplementation should be considered.

DISCLOSURE

The authors have nothing to disclose.

REFERENCES

1. Tabolli S, Bergamo F, Alessandroni L, et al. Quality of life and psychological problems of patients with oral mucosal disease in dermatological practice. Dermatology (Basel) 2009;218(4):314–20.
2. Nevalainen MJ, Närhi TO, Ainamo A. Oral mucosal lesions and oral hygiene habits in the home-living elderly. J Oral Rehabil 1997;24(5):332–7.
3. Suliman NM, Johannessen AC, Ali RW, et al. Influence of oral mucosal lesions and oral symptoms on oral health related quality of life in dermatological patients: a cross sectional study in Sudan. BMC Oral Health 2012;12:19.
4. Rashid H, Lamberts A, Diercks GFH, et al. Oral lesions in autoimmune bullous diseases: an overview of clinical characteristics and diagnostic algorithm. Am J Clin Dermatol 2019;20:847–61.
5. Fatahzadeh M, Radfar L, Sirois DA. Dental care of patients with autoimmune vesiculobullous diseases: case reports and literature review. Quintessence Int 2006;37(10):777–87.
6. Giannobile WV, Braun TM, Caplis AK, et al. Patient stratification for preventive care in dentistry. J Dent Res 2013;92(8):694–701.
7. Radfar L, Ahmadabadi RE, Masood F, et al. Biological therapy and dentistry: a review paper. Oral Surg Oral Med Oral Pathol Oral Radiol 2015;120(5):594–601.
8. Carbone M, Goss E, Carrozzo M, et al. Systemic and topical corticosteroid treatment of oral lichen planus: a comparative study with long-term follow-up. J Oral Pathol Med 2003;32:323–9.
9. Patil P, Jain H, Mishra V, et al. Sarcoidosis: an update for the oral health care provider. Journal of Cranio-Maxillary Diseases 2015;4(1):69–75.
10. Wang Y, Li C, Yuan H, et al. Rubber dam isolation for restorative treatment in dental patients. Cochrane Database Syst Rev 2016;(9):CD009858.
11. Ucak O, Haytac M, Akkaya M. Iatrogenic Trauma to Oral Tissues. J Periodontol 2005;76:1793–7.
12. Reichart PA. Oral lichen planus and dental implants. Report of 3 cases. Int J Oral Maxillofac Surg 2006;35(3):237–40.
13. Elad S, Epstein JB, Von bültzingslöwen I, et al. Topical immunomodulators for management of oral mucosal conditions, a systematic review; Part II: miscellaneous agents. Expert Opin Emerg Drugs 2011;16(1):183–202.
14. Kulkarni R, Payne AS, Werth VP, et al. Custom dental trays with topical corticosteroids for management of gingival lesions of mucous membrane pemphigoid. Int J Dermatol 2020;59(6):e211–3.
15. Goldman KE. Dental management of patients with bone marrow and solid organ transplantation. Dent Clin North Am 2006;50(4):659–76, viii.
16. Meier JK, Wolff D, Pavletic S, et al. Oral chronic graft-versus-host disease: report from the International

Consensus Conference on clinical practice in cGVHD. Clin Oral Investig 2011;15(2):127–39.

17. Goldstein BG, Goldstein AO. Dellavalle/Section Editor RP, Levy/Section Editor ML, Corona/Deputy Editor R. Topical corticosteroids: use and adverse effects. UpToDate. 2020. Available at: https://www.uptodate.com/contents/topical-corticosteroids-use-and-adverse-effects/print. Accessed February 24, 2020.

18. Thorburn D, Ferguson M. Topical corticosteroids and lesions of the oral mucosa. Adv Drug Deliv Rev 1994;13(1–2):135–49.

19. Feiwel M, James VH, Barnett ES. Effect of potent topical steroids on plasma-cortisol levels of infants and children with eczema. Lancet 1969;1(7593):485–7.

20. Guin JD. Contact sensitivity to topical corticosteroids. J Am Acad Dermatol 1984;10(5 Pt 1):773–82.

21. Davis MDP, el-Azhary RA, Farmer SA. Results of patch testing to a corticosteroid series: a retrospective review of 1188 patients during 6 years at Mayo Clinic. J Am Acad Dermatol 2007;56(6):921–7.

22. Hengge UR, Ruzicka T, Schwartz RA, et al. Adverse effects of topical glucocorticosteroids. J Am Acad Dermatol 2006;54(1):1–15 [quiz: 16].

23. Seo P. Furst/Section Editor D, Curtis/Deputy Editor MR. Mycophenolate: overview of use and adverse effects in the treatment of rheumatic diseases. UpToDate. 2019. Available at: https://www.uptodate.com/contents/mycophenolate-overview-of-use-and-adverse-effects-in-the-treatment-of-rheumatic-diseases/print. Accessed February 23, 2020.

24. Clayton R, Chaudhry S, Ali I, et al. Mucosal (oral and vulval) lichen planus in women: are angiotensin-converting enzyme inhibitors protective, and beta-blockers and non-steroidal anti-inflammatory drugs associated with the condition? Clin Exp Dermatol 2010;35(4):384–7.

25. Ciarrocca KN, Greenberg MS. A retrospective study of the management of oral mucous membrane pemphigoid with dapsone. Oral Surg Oral Med Oral Pathol Oral Radiol Endod 1999;88(2):159–63.

26. Coleman MD. Dapsone: modes of action, toxicity and possible strategies for increasing patient tolerance. Br J Dermatol 1993;129(5):507–13.

27. Sapadin AN, Fleischmajer R. Tetracyclines: nonantibiotic properties and their clinical implications. J Am Acad Dermatol 2006;54(2):258–65.

28. Sánchez AR, Rogers RS, Sheridan PJ. Tetracycline and other tetracycline-derivative staining of the teeth and oral cavity. Int J Dermatol 2004;43(10):709–15.

29. The Effect of Cytochrome P450 Metabolism on Drug Response, Interactions, and Adverse Effects - American Family Physician. Available at: https://www.aafp.org/afp/2007/0801/p391.html. Accessed April 27, 2020.

30. Katz HI, Gupta AK. Oral antifungal drug interactions. Dermatol Clin 2003;21(3):543–63.

31. Bagg A, Dunphy CH. Immunosuppressive and immunomodulatory therapy-associated lymphoproliferative disorders. Semin Diagn Pathol 2013;30(2):102–12.

32. Yuan A, Woo S-B. Adverse drug events in the oral cavity. Oral Surg Oral Med Oral Pathol Oral Radiol 2015;119(1):35–47.

33. Berger TG, Duvic M, Van Voorhees AS, et al, American Academy of Dermatology Association Task Force. The use of topical calcineurin inhibitors in dermatology: safety concerns. Report of the American Academy of Dermatology Association Task Force. J Am Acad Dermatol 2006;54(5):818–23.

34. Tennis P, Gelfand JM, Rothman KJ. Evaluation of cancer risk related to atopic dermatitis and use of topical calcineurin inhibitors. Br J Dermatol 2011;165(3):465–73.

35. Bongartz T, Sutton AJ, Sweeting MJ, et al. Anti-TNF antibody therapy in rheumatoid arthritis and the risk of serious infections and malignancies: systematic review and meta-analysis of rare harmful effects in randomized controlled trials. JAMA 2006;295(19):2275–85.

36. Baecklund E, Backlin C, Iliadou A, et al. Characteristics of diffuse large B cell lymphomas in rheumatoid arthritis. Arthritis Rheum 2006;54(12):3774–81.

37. Niwa Y, Terashima T, Sumi H. Topical application of the immunosuppressant tacrolimus accelerates carcinogenesis in mouse skin. Br J Dermatol 2003;149(5):960–7.

38. Mabrouk D, Gürcan HM, Keskin DB, et al. Association between cancer and immunosuppressive therapy–analysis of selected studies in pemphigus and pemphigoid. Ann Pharmacother 2010;44(11):1770–6.

39. Stoopler ET, Sollecito TP. Oral mucosal diseases: evaluation and management. Med Clin North Am 2014;98(6):1323–52.

40. McCreary CE, McCartan BE. Clinical management of oral lichen planus. Br J Oral Maxillofac Surg 1999;37(5):338–43.

41. Farah CS, Lynch N, McCullough MJ. Oral fungal infections: an update for the general practitioner. Aust Dent J 2010;55(Suppl 1):48–54.

42. Muzyka BC, Epifanio RN. Update on oral fungal infections. Dent Clin North Am 2013;57(4):561–81.

43. Dowd FJ. Saliva and dental caries. Dent Clin North Am 1999;43(4):579–97.

Moving?

Make sure your subscription moves with you!

To notify us of your new address, find your **Clinics Account Number** (located on your mailing label above your name), and contact customer service at:

Email: journalscustomerservice-usa@elsevier.com

800-654-2452 (subscribers in the U.S. & Canada)
314-447-8871 (subscribers outside of the U.S. & Canada)

Fax number: 314-447-8029

Elsevier Health Sciences Division
Subscription Customer Service
3251 Riverport Lane
Maryland Heights, MO 63043

*To ensure uninterrupted delivery of your subscription, please notify us at least 4 weeks in advance of move.

Printed and bound by CPI Group (UK) Ltd, Croydon, CR0 4YY

03/10/2024

01040370-0015